MW01348567

# ANYONE CAN
# DIY
## — WITH —
## Essential Oils

## AMY WALQUIST, RN, BSN

Copyright © 2018 Amy Walquist. Book and cover design copyright © 2018 Growing Healthy Homes LLC¨. All rights reserved. No part of this book may be reproduced, stored, or transmitted in any form or by any means, electronic, mechanical, photocopying or recording without the express written permission of the author and publisher.

ISBN: 978-0-9988534-6-8
Printed in the United States of America
First printing.

Growing Healthy Homes LLC
P.O. Box 3154
Bartlesville, OK 74006

To obtain additional copies of this book, please visit www.GrowingHealthyHomes.com.

Disclaimer: The information contained in this book has not been evaluated by the FDA and is intended for educational purposes only. The author is not a physician and therefore is not authorized to diagnose or treat for specific sicknesses or disease. Information provided is based on the author's personal research and experiences with Young Living¨ Essential Oils. If you are under the care of a health care provider for any disease, it is recommended that you discuss adding Young Living¨ Essential Oils to your health care regime before starting to use them.

# Special thanks

Robert, my first and only love, thank you for supporting me in all my dreams, even when they keep me up at night. You are a perfect example of selfless love. I am forever yours.

My children: Andrew, Brittany and Daniel; thank you for supporting Mom in her new career and calling. You are, and always will be, your Dad's and my greatest accomplishments.

Jennifer and Brooke, my oily sisters who loved me through the writing of this book, to thank you here is just not enough. This book wouldn't exist without your support and encouragement.

Karen Hopkins, I am thankful that God brought our paths together in a way only He could. Thank you for your mentorship with the revision of this book. I am truly grateful.

To these and more who have supported me in following my dreams:

> *"All our dreams can come true if we have
> the courage to pursue them."*
>
> ~ *Walt Disney*

# Dedication

My journey since discovering Young Living Essential Oils and incorporating essential oils into the lives of my family members makes me feel like I am one step closer to becoming a "Proverbs 31 woman".

I share this scripture not as a tribute to myself, but to *you*, the **Mother** reading this book. You, my friend are the gatekeeper of your home. You have the power and ability to change generations by taking the road less traveled. This life can be challenging and many things are outside of your control, but as the woman of the home, you choose the food, products, and health care options for your family. Choose well. Live well. I can't wait to hear your story! I am cheering for you.

*Proverbs 31: 27-31*
*27 She watches over the ways of her household,*
*And does not eat the bread of idleness.*
*28 Her children rise up and call her blessed;*
*Her husband also, and he praises her:*
*29 "Many daughters have done well,*
*But you excel them all."*
*30 Charm is deceitful and beauty is passing,*
*But a woman who fears the Lord, she shall be praised.*
*31 Give her of the fruit of her hands,*
*And let her own works praise her in the gates.*

# table of Contents

# Introduction

My name is Amy, and I have been married to my best friend, Robert, for over 20 years. We have been truly blessed with the privilege of raising our three kids, all of whom are now young adults. God has sent us down paths we never would have chosen, but we have learned so much along the way. We wouldn't change our story for anything. We feel as if we have grown up together, working out love, parenting, finances, careers, and marriage.

I graduated in 1994 with a bachelor's degree in nursing. I have worked in the nursing field in some capacity for nearly all of the years since that time, only taking a few years off to stay at home with my kiddos. In the medical field, my first love was pediatrics, and I have spent the majority of my career working in that specialty. I have worked in office nursing, phone triage, school nursing and floor nursing.

In 2008, I was working at a job that I loved when I started volunteering for a non-profit pregnancy resource center in the Kansas City area. That decision changed the path of my life. I became passionate about my work at this center, believing I was making a difference in the community. This ministry work is still vitally important to me because it is part of my life's calling.

In the fall of 2013, I was introduced to the world of essential oils, and everything was turned upside-down. I first fell in love with the oils themselves. With all those aromas and amazingly powerful testimonies, what's not to love? Although my sweetie was a reluctant oil user in the beginning, he has become the biggest oil fan of all. He talks with everyone who will listen about his genuine love for Young Living Essential Oils.

Next came the knowledge that I was unknowingly using toxic products on my husband, my kiddos, and myself every day. I learned that commercial deodorants contain aluminum, a naturally occurring metal. I found out that this toxin has links to very serious illnesses to which I don't want to expose my family. (If it is true, why take a chance?) This was my "Y" in the road. Everyone is faced with them – those moments when you look back on your life and realize that you need to decide. Those times when you know you need to acknowledge your mistakes, and then you choose to CHANGE.

In my case, this meant I couldn't continue to purchase very inexpensive cleaners, deodorants, shampoos, and conditioners that were causing harm to us. So, I began to make changes. Slowly, one or two items at a time, I started making my own replacement products that were 100% chemically safe. To our surprise, most of my DIY products were just as effective as their chemical-laden counterparts, if not more so. Of course, there was some trial and error, and a few things even got pitched along the way, but my overall experience with making our own personal care products and cleaners has been an enormous success!

I recommend starting with a few new things per month and adding on gradually from there. Start with something relatively simple and exchange that item throughout the whole house. A few good baby steps to begin with are hand soap, hand purifier, and all-purpose cleaners. As time goes on, you can tackle some more involved items like lotion and bar soap. Follow a step-by-step approach and have confidence that you can do this!

The ingredients for most products are basic, and I am going to walk you through with simple instructions. Many of the items that you will need to purchase can be used for multiple DIY items. Remember, doing the same thing you've always done may be easier, but the road less traveled is the correct one many times in life. Let's get started today on your clean, non-toxic lifestyle.

You'll never regret it, I promise.

*Amy Walquist*

# Why DIY?

Early in my nursing career, the pediatrics group I worked at did a fantastic job of teaching me about the overuse of antibiotics and their adverse effects. You see, the overuse of antibiotics has a devastating effect on the health of individuals, as well as a negative impact on society as a whole. When we introduce an antibiotic into our system, it kills all bacteria – the good and the bad. The end result is a compromised immune system that is more susceptible to the next infection that comes along. This means that infections become harder to treat and oftentimes, take longer to conquer.

All of this can be attributed to the ill effects of the overuse of antibiotics. This knowledge led me to avoid medications for my family and myself whenever possible. Before essential oils, we tried lots of home remedies, some successful and many unsuccessful. My kids used to say that I was always trying to use honey, apple cider vinegar, and coconut oil for everything.

In 2013, we had some minor issues in our family, and we were trying to address them through natural products and a controlled diet without much success. My daughter was struggling with typical teenage acne and mild heartburn. The acne was a particularly sensitive issue for me because I had struggled with my own complexion for years, and I didn't want my kids to struggle with it. However, I was also unwilling to go the conventional route with my daughter. We had been seeing a dermatologist and had tried a few of the milder creams, but we were not pleased with the lack of results. I was not willing to medicate her with long-term antibiotics in order to "potentially" improve her skin.

It was about this time when my sister introduced me to Young Living Essential Oils (YLEO). She had begun successfully using them with her family and encouraged me to try them. I first invested in YLEOs for the acne and mild heartburn issues that my daughter struggled with, but then I realized that there were literally thousands of uses for them. They are actually highly beneficial to our bodies. I was hooked, and our success continued.

Now, don't misunderstand me, it wasn't entirely a smooth transition. We had some verbal fallout over using oils. My boys, particularly my eldest, who knows so much about the world, were strongly against the use of oils in our home. Even my darling hubby initially called the oils my "voodoo kit". I ignored the criticism and pressed on, knowing I had found a gold mine. They soon began to criticize less and ask for YLEOs more. I knew that they had finally seen the light.

My next step was acknowledging that most of the products in our bathrooms and under the kitchen sink were literally *toxic*. At that time in our lives, purchasing expensive organic or "green" products wasn't an option, so I started down the DIY road. We began to transition to using homemade products for our everyday needs, as well as replacing store bought health and beauty products.

We have been blessed enormously by the using essential oils. We are healthier and feel better than ever. Our home is much greener and more toxin-free. I love that when I look at products in my shower and under my counters, I KNOW every ingredient in them and where they came from! I love that I am living similarly to the way my great-grandmother did with a few cleaning products and soaps that I have made myself. This process has included a significant investment of time, money and research, but it has been worth it, hands down.

Now, when my hubby and I walk near the laundry aisle at the big box store, we instantly feel the need to leave; the harsh odors are offensive to our bodies. We are so accustomed to pure, natural, God-made smells that the synthetic smells are offensive. This change has been one of the most dramatic of our lives!

# Ingredient Snob

When transitioning to toxic-free products, it is important to research and check ingredients carefully. You will need to become an ingredient snob in order to eliminate the "nasties" from your lifestyle. What can be so wrong with products that our government has deemed "safe" for our use? Haven't they evaluated, tested, and approved these ingredients that are labeled as *safe*? Unfortunately, the answer is NO.

The cosmetic, cleaning and self-care product industry is big business! Billions of dollars are made from people trying to smell and look good. Household cleaning is another multi-billion-dollar industry. With the advancement of time and technology, more and more products are continually showing up on grocery store shelves. These products contain more fragrances, more chemicals and more additives to supposedly make them work better. I am fairly sure that my great-grandma didn't need 42 cleaners in her home. I believe she used just a few cleaners for her entire home, and those products didn't have a list of ingredients as long as the genealogy of Jesus.

There are many reasons to avoid using the chemicals talked about here, generally recognized as safe (GRAS) by the FDA. Many are endocrine disruptors that cause damage to major organs in the body, including the liver, kidneys, thyroid, and brain. Many are skin irritants. Some are known carcinogens: chemicals that cause cancer. Others are also commonly used as engine degreasers, floor cleaners, and pesticides. The list of the consequences related to using these chemicals goes on and on.

When I was in college, I worked for a major chemical company (ironic, I know). I worked all summer with Material Safety Data Sheets (MSDS), which are published by the government. This information gives the proper handling instructions for different chemicals so that every company using a particular chemical follows the same standardized precautions. If you were to look up the MSDS on many ingredients in common household cleaning products, you would see that it is REQUIRED for workers to wear protective HAZMAT gear when handling these chemicals! What?! By the way, this same junk is also present in smaller quantities in our health and beauty products, even those formulated for babies and children. Many of these chemicals are illegal in other countries but are currently allowed in the USA.

## HARMFUL CHEMICALS FOUND IN COMMON HOUSEHOLD PRODUCTS

I am sure you have noticed that the labels on chemical household products are often confusing and misleading. Many chemicals have several different names. Once a chemical is proven harmful, manufactures are expert at changing or inventing new names for it to deceive consumers. That is another reason why it is vitally important that we continue to research the ingredients in the products we use.

It would be impossible to list all the harmful chemicals that are present in traditional household and personal care products; however, I will list a few of the most commonly found offenders here. If you have time, go check out some stuff lingering in your cabinets. If you want to do more thorough research, refer to some of the resources listed at the end of the book.

## Aluminum

**Other names:** alum, alumen
**Found in:** deodorants, antacids, shampoos, cosmetics, lotions
**Risks/Dangers:** linked to breast cancer, Alzheimer's disease, epilepsy, dementia, ADD, and chronic fatigue syndrome

## Fluoride

**Other names:** acidulated phosphate fluoride, atomic number 9, calcarea fluorica, fluorophosphates, monofluorophosphate, MFP
**Found in:** toothpastes, mouthwash, and other dental products
**Risks/Dangers:** developmental neurotoxin; linked to birth defects; possible toxic carcinogen; leads to lower IQ in children; disrupts thyroid function

## Formaldehyde

**Other names:** formalin, formic aldehyde, methanediol, methanol, methyl aldehyde, methylene glycol, methylene oxide
**Found in:** cosmetics, fabric softeners, dishwashing soap
**Risks/Dangers:** known carcinogen

## Parabens

**Other names:** methylparaben, any ingredient containing "ethyl", "butyl", "methyl", "propyl"
**Found in:** skin care products, lotions, deodorants
**Risks/Dangers:** endocrine disruptor; linked to developmental and reproductive toxicity

## Phthalates

**Other names:** DBP, DEP, DEHP, DMP, BzBP
**Found in:** deodorants, sprays, lotions and household cleaners
**Risks/Dangers:** endocrine disruptor; linked to birth defects and obesity

**Petroleum** – derived from crude oil
  **Other names:** petrolatum, mineral oil jelly, paraffin jelly, soft paraffin
  **Found in:** deodorants and other health care products
  **Risks/Dangers:** skin irritant; possible carcinogen; classified as a xenoestrogen (hormone disruptor)

**Propylene glycol**
  **Other names:** propanediol, methyl ethyl glycol, MEG, methylethylene glycol, PG 12
  **Found in:** moisturizers, sunscreens, cosmetics, conditioners, shampoos, hairsprays
  **Risks/Dangers:** skin irritant; respiratory irritant; potentially toxic to the liver and kidneys; linked to heart disease and neurological issues

**Sodium lauryl sulfate**
  **Other names:** SLS, sodium dodecyl sulfate
  **Found in:** shampoos and soaps
  **Risks/Dangers:** developmental/reproductive toxin; irritant to those with asthma/allergies; skin irritant; possible carcinogen

**Toluene** – restricted in European Union
  **Other names:** benzene, methylbenzene, toluol, phenylmethane
  Found in: dyes, detergents, cosmetics, cleaning products
  **Risks/Dangers:** developmental and reproductive toxin; skin irritant; known carcinogen

**Triclosan** – restricted in Canada and Japan; regulated as a pesticide
  **Other names:** Ultra-Fresh, Irgacare, viv-20, Microban, Biofresh, Amicor
  **Found in:** antibacterial hand soaps, dishwashing liquids,

laundry soaps, fabric softeners, disinfectants, kitchen wipes, deodorants, cosmetics, toothpastes

**Risks/Dangers:** environmental hazard; skin irritant; reproductive and developmental toxin; possible carcinogen; hormone disruptor; causes antibiotic resistance

## FRAGRANCES

Fragrances deserve special mention. "Fragrance" is a very general term permitted by the FDA to include thousands of different chemicals. When fragrance is added to a product, the consumer has no idea what it actually is. Many fragrances are known skin irritants and/or have negative respiratory effects with ingredients that can aggravate allergic and asthmatic reactions. Fragrance can refer to chemicals that mimic natural smells (which is cheapest and most profitable for the manufacturer) that may also be cancer-causing agents.

Most often, any fragrance added to products indicates unsafe chemicals. Why is this so? The FDA believes that forcing companies marketing self-care products to disclose EVERY single ingredient in a particular product means they will be giving up their trade secrets. So in order to protect the business interests of the chemical companies, we are not given full disclosure on what is in the products we use on our bodies and those of our loved ones. Fragrance, or perfume, is found in nearly every household cleaning and personal care product.

## WHAT'S THE BIG DEAL ANYWAY?

This list is just a drop-in-the-bucket regarding the harmful ingredients that are commonly found in everyday household products in the United States. The U.S. government has grandfathered in a great number of the chemicals used in household products because of a law passed in 1976 called the

Toxic Substance Control Act. This means that many chemicals have not been adequately tested, and their safety (or lack thereof) is completely unknown. The FDA's reasoning to list many chemicals as safe, even without proper research or testing, is simply because they have been used in America for over 100 years with no proof through research that there are connections to serious sickness, disease, or cancer. Do you really want to use these products in your home?

Another important point is that even though something is labeled as organic, green, environmentally safe, naturally derived, or natural, it may not actually be any of those things! I remember when I brought home a huge jug of "green" dish soap and looked at the ingredients. The very first one listed was sodium lauryl sulfate, which as previously noted, has been implicated in developmental and or reproductive toxicity, as an irritant to those with asthma or allergies, a skin irritant, and a possible carcinogen.

There is a better way, my friends. I am sure I have convinced you by now, so off on the adventure we go!

# What Are Essential Oils?

**HISTORICAL USE**

You may think that essential oils are just useful for fragrance. I used to think that as well. Early in my oily journey, I realized that there was a lot more to essential oils than what I thought. The use of essential oils actually pre-dates biblical times. In fact, evidence shows that essential oils were used thousands of years before Jesus walked the earth and were commonly used for every ailment that people encountered. The Bible tells us that frankincense and myrrh were even brought to Jesus as a boy. Frankincense held more value at that time than did money.

**HOW ESSENTIAL OILS ARE MADE**

Essential oils are derived from plants, trees, flowers, roots, and shrubs. It is critically important that the highest quality seeds from the healthiest plants are used, and that they are cultivated in healthy soil that hasn't been contaminated with chemicals. Most essential oils today are produced using steam distillation. It is a complicated process and is not easily replicated. Vast research has been done to determine the exact time when each type of plant is ready to be distilled in order to ensure its full compliment of chemical constituents will be in the resulting oil. The plant is cut and distilled when it is at its peak a point in time that is different for each and every plant species. The temperature and length of time necessary for proper distillation varies for each plant as well. Once distilled, the scientific folks carefully perform extensive testing to verify the chemical compounds have remained intact. Each Young Living farm has a testing laboratory on site for this purpose.

When the essential oil leaves the farm, it is sent to the Young Living warehouse where it undergoes even further testing before bottling. My favorite part is when the oil is bottled and all of the inherent properties and fabulous goodness that were keeping the plant vibrant and healthy are made available to us. When a plant is cultivated under ideal growing conditions in the very best soil and is distilled with the greatest care, we reap many amazing healing properties from the resulting essential oil.

As you can see, essential oils are so much more than aromatic liquids. They smell amazing and have fabulous properties that support each and every system in our bodies. They are, in my opinion, the most powerful tools available to us today to support optimal health.

## HOW TO USE ESSENTIAL OILS

In the essential oil world, there are historically three different models of application: German, English, and French. The German model focuses strictly on aromatherapy, or the inhalation of essential oils. The English model recommends heavy dilution and topical use through massage. The French model encourages neat, or undiluted, application and ingestion of pure, therapeutic essential oils. Young Living Essential Oils follows the French model, and YL oils are suitable for all methods of usage: topical, aromatic, and internal. My family has had great success using oils in all of these different ways.

*(Note: I would never recommend the ingestion of an essential oil brand other than Young Living.)*

## ESSENTIAL OIL REGULATION (OR LACK THEREOF)

There are tons of low-quality oils available on the market. With the rise in popularity of essential oils in recent years, the industry has naturally become flooded. Because the Federal Drug Administration (FDA) does not regulate the cultivation, production, or marketing of essential oils in the United States, the labeling can be very deceptive. In fact, there are no quality standards for the authentication of essential oils in place. This means that it is entirely possible to purchase a bottle of essential oil that is labeled "pure, therapeutic grade" that has been adulterated. These oils are often diluted with fillers or additives, like a carrier oil, alcohol, and/or synthetic fragrance. What's even worse is that oils don't even have to be natural to be labeled as such. Scientists have figured out ways to re-create chemical compounds found in plants to create completely synthetic essential oils, and these can be labeled as therapeutic, just as natural oils can.

## BEWARE OF IMITATORS

It is surprising how many products labeled essential oils are actually synthetic (created in a laboratory). These imitators may smell good to the untrained nose – especially if you have been subjected to decades of artificial smells – and yet be completely toxic and harmful to your body. Recently, I found an old bottle of an off-brand essential oil in my crafting supplies and remembered scenting candles for Christmas gifts one year. What that bottle actually contained was a synthetic fragrance that mimicked the aroma of a true essential oil.

I have noticed another significant change from my pre-oily life: I used to love going into bath and body stores with a lot of fragrances. If I venture into one of those stores now, I instantly feel pressure in my head and want to leave. My body – and more importantly, my limbic system – is aware that these are not natural smells and is repelled by them.

Speaking of toxins, it is also important to evaluate the use of artificial smells, aromas, and sprays in your home. Before YL, I had so many candles in my home; they were in my bathrooms, kitchen, and even our bedroom. They were among the first things that I ditched when I began to learn that the indoor air quality was toxic because of the things that I chose to bring into it. Additional offenders include plug-ins, sprays, and other air fresheners. You simply do not want to be breathing in those chemicals! These items can easily be replaced with a high quality cold air diffuser and essential oils.

So when shopping for essential oils, it is critically important that you do your research to ensure that you are getting true therapeutic grade essential oils. After all, you are going to all of this trouble to remove toxins, so why compromise on your essential oils?

## CONSIDER THE SOURCE

The way your oils are handled, from the time they are just seeds filled with potential to when they are sealed in bottles, is of utmost importance. Choosing the right company from which to purchase your oils is the most important decision you will make during this journey.

Based on my research, I believe that the majority of essential oils in the marketplace are adulterated or synthetic. I count myself blessed. When I was first introduced to Young Living Essential Oils, I really didn't know anything about oils. I am grateful that when I found oils, I jumped on board with the world leader in the essential oil industry. The founder and owner, Gary Young, does not believe in adulterating (adding chemicals that are foreign to the plant) or extending the oils with alcohol.

If you are wondering how you can be sure you are purchasing the highest quality essential oils, I encourage you to do your own research. You will need to do some detective work and learn about the company and how they obtain their oils:

- Do they own their own farms?
- Do they oversee every farm and hold them to rigorous standards of planting and cultivating?
- Are they setting the industry standard for quality and purity?
- Do they distill their own oils?
- Do they subject every batch of essential oil to thorough testing, including third-party testing, to ensure quality and purity?
- Are you able to visit their farms and watch them distill the oils at any time?
- Are they leading the industry in essential oils and conducting world-changing research?

To each of these questions, the answer is YES for Young Living.

## CHOOSE THE BEST

Young Living offers a guarantee to its customers called the Seed to Seal® promise. This is a personal promise that they will maintain the STRICTEST quality control to ensure that Young Living customers get the best product possible. This doesn't just apply to the essential oils that Young Living produces, but to every product that they sell. Young Living employs over 50 scientists and has some of the most sophisticated laboratories in the world. With Young Living products, you don't have to be a label-reader because the ingredients found in YL oils, supplements, and other products are guaranteed safe for you and your family. The Young Living Seed to Seal® promise ensures that you will receive only the purist and very best essential oils and other products, no question.

Young Living also offers a line of oils specifically labeled for internal use. The Vitality™ line was created because the FDA has certain categories that every product must fit into, and it does not allow for a product to be labeled for multiple categories. Since many YL oils have dietary and topical/aromatic uses, they developed a labeling system to differentiate between the two categories.

## MORE THAN JUST ESSENTIAL OILS

At first, I just wanted to use the oils because they smelled good, but I soon began a life transformation that involved using Young Living oils aromatically, topically and internally. As I became educated on how to use YLEOs, I exchanged conventional products I was using for products that are infused with YLEOs, one at a time. I literally started pitching things out of my house by the box-full: medications, creams, lotions, hair products, deodorants, etc. It was a dump fest! Some things I pitched even before I had a YL replacement product for it.

Here's a shout-out to those who are still a bit overwhelmed with the concept of DIY-ing everything in your home. Young Living began as an essential oil company and has grown into a health and wellness company that offers more than 600 products and is still growing. YL has the largest selection of pure plant-based oils of any company in the world. Did you know that YL also offers a dental care line, self-care products (shampoo, conditioner, shave cream, massage oils, lotion, etc.), skin care, make-up, supplements, cleaning products, baby and kids lines, and even a fantastic pet line? As I explained earlier, because of my family budget and the fact that I love making things myself, I began by mostly making DIY products using my YLEOs. Now my family uses more Young Living products and fewer of my DIY concoctions. However, there are certain DIY items I will never stop making because I love them and enjoy the process.

# Fill Your toolbox

You are going to need some supplies to get started with DIY. I will provide a simple list of things that I recommend as you begin your journey towards a healthier, toxin-free home. You don't have to purchase all of the items right away. Choose where you want to begin, and purchase what you need to get started. You will find that many of the items are already in your home.

Health food stores and organic grocery stores are great places to shop for supplies. Some bulk stores also carry a few goodies. I order most of the harder-to-find ingredients from Amazon. Remember, you will need to make an initial investment in the beginning, but you will get used to wheeling right past the cleaning and self-care aisles at your local grocery store, which will eventually pay off. It's called transfer spending. Spend a bit here instead of there. For my budget-conscious family, it all balanced out in the end.

As you shop for supplies, remember to look carefully at all labels. Don't assume that manufactures don't sneak fragrances or other chemicals in with "natural" ingredients. When I began my journey, I couldn't believe how many items were advertised as containing pure ingredients but had other things in them. Don't worry; it will get easier. Once you find your favorite stores and become familiar with safe-to-use products and labels, it's easy-peasy.

One decision for you to make in the beginning is whether or not you want to insist on organic ingredients. I try to use mostly organic whenever possible; however, I did not in the beginning.

I had a lot of changes to make and a lot to learn. I was in the process of learning the industry and their labeling strategies. You will learn along the way as well, so don't condemn yourself when you discover the truth. If you choose organic, certain items will often be harder to find. Much of my purchasing is done online simply for the sake of ease.

**By simply making your own DIY items, you are miles ahead of the pack! I love organic products and try to purchase as many of them as I can for my family. However, if it's not in your budget, then pat yourself on the back just for making the change to DIY, organic or not.**

The list below is rather extensive and covers most of what you would need in order to create nearly all of the recipes in this book. If you want to start slowly, select specific recipes and purchase only what you need. Most recipes only require 3-5 ingredients.

*Note: I chose not to include supplies for making bar soap here because it is the most difficult DIY project listed in this book. When you are ready for soap-making, consult the list in that chapter (pp 89).*

## INGREDIENTS LIST

Almond oil
Aloe vera juice (no additives)
Apple cider vinegar (I like Bragg's®)
Arrowroot powder
Baking soda (aluminum-free)
Beeswax pellets or crystals
Castile soap (I like Dr. Bronner's®)
Castor oil
Citric acid

Cocoa butter
Coconut milk
Coconut oil, cold pressed and unrefined
Cornstarch
Cream of tartar
Distilled water
Epsom salts
Extra virgin olive oil
Flour
Grapeseed oil

Jojoba oil
Salt, fine
Shea butter
Sugar, brown and white (for sugar scrubs)
Vegetable glycerin
Vinegar
Vitamin E oil
Washing soda
Witch hazel
100% wool yarn – for dryer balls

## SUPPLIES

15 mL bottles (recycled essential oil bottles)
Dropper bottle (small, dark glass, for cuticle oil)
Foaming hand soap containers (empty and clean)
Glass bottles (various sizes, preferably dark-colored glass)
Glass jars (I like to use 4 oz. glass canning jars and white lids)
Glass spray bottles (various sizes, preferably dark-colored glass)
Labels
Lip balm tubes or small bead containers
Measuring cups, spoons, spatulas
Microfiber cloths
Plastic spray bottles (large, for cleaning products)
Soap molds (for lotion bars)
Stainless steel roller tops

## YOUNG LIVING ESSENTIAL OILS

My list of DIY essential oils is extensive. As you experiment, you will learn which oils your family favors. This brief list is intended to be a starting point. You will surely want to add to your essential oil collection as you gain experience.

## AMY'S TOP 10

Cedarwood
Lavender
Lemon
Lemongrass
Orange
Peppermint
Purification®
Stress Away™
Tea Tree
Thieves®

# Beginner tips

Let me start by saying that I have never been more confident in anything that I have chosen for my family than Young Living Essential Oils. I could write another entire book on the positive impact, testimonies, and crazy awesome successes that we (myself, my immediate family, and my extended family) have had with Young Living oils and products.

Using essential oils safely is really pretty basic: use common sense and follow a few simple guidelines. Keep in mind that each of our bodies is unique and can react differently to any substance, natural or synthetic; however, there is simply no need to fear when beginning to use essential oils, as long as you are using pure therapeutic essential oils.

I believe with every fiber of my being that essential oils are a God-made gift from our Creator. Each time I approach a challenge, I approach it with this in mind. Man-made synthetic substances are much more difficult for our bodies to metabolize and process. God programmed essential oils to be intelligent, complex substances that "know" what our bodies need and enhance our bodies' ability to heal themselves.

As I begin to address a few general guidelines for beginning oilers, be aware that these tips will become second nature to you. You won't always have to look up which oils are photosensitive, the best application method, or even dilution ratios, because you will become more and more confident with your oils. You can do this, and I am happy to cheer you on as you do!

## START SLOWLY

I want you to be successful with your oils! In the beginning, apply one oil or blend at a time, and allow your body time to adjust to the oils. You may experience mild detox effects, and this is a normal and beneficial part of the process. As you eliminate more toxins and your body becomes used to the oils, you may begin using more oils at one time. Eventually, you will adjust to new aromas, even those that you may not have loved at first.

TIP: I have learned that an oil that smells bad to me is usually an oil that my body needs. Apply that oil to your feet and cover with cotton socks. Eventually it will help your body release toxins, and the smell won't bother you anymore.

## DILUTION

It is sometimes advisable to dilute an essential oil with a fatty oil, such as extra-virgin olive oil, almond oil, coconut oil, or Young Living's V-6™ Vegetable Oil Complex. Dilution is often a good idea when you are first starting out. Dilution slows down the absorption rate of the essential oil but does not affect the efficacy, so go ahead and dilute. As you become a seasoned oiler, your body may require less dilution. When my family first started out, we diluted much of the time, and oftentimes, we applied our oils on our hands or feet. Now, we rarely dilute and rarely have any skin sensitivities.

Some reasons for dilution are to cover a larger surface area or because some oils are considered "hot", meaning they may feel warm to the skin when applied undiluted. Young Living's V-6™ carrier oil is a blend of six different vegetable-based oils. This non-greasy blend is a highly effective carrier oil and is a favorite in our home. You can use other fatty oils listed above, but keep in mind that you will have to seek out a quality source, and sadly labeling cannot always be trusted. You can be assured that V-6™ is processed with only the highest quality carrier oils that are never subjected to harsh chemicals during processing.

## SUN SENSITIVITY

Citrus oils can increase your sensitivity to the sun when used topically. When using citrus oils on your skin, stay out of direct sunlight for 24-48 hours. One exception: although tangerine is a citrus oil, it does not cause photosensitivity.

## EYES AND EARS

When using essential oils near the eyes and ears, it is best to proceed with caution. Oils can be diluted and placed around the bone of the outer ears. Alternatively, you may dilute with a carrier oil, place on an unbleached cotton ball, and rest the cotton ball inside the ear. The eyes are especially sensitive to essential oils. It is rarely ever necessary to do more than apply a diluted essential oil around the bone of the eyes. As a seasoned oiler, I can assure you that at one time or another, you will accidentally get essential oil in your eye. It will sting a bit but thankfully is easy to remedy. Simply add a bit of carrier oil to the area; NEVER use water. (Since oil and water don't mix, water will actually intensify the burning.) It is best to avoid the use of "hot" oils altogether when using near the eyes and ears (oregano, cinnamon, Thieves®, lemongrass etc.).

## PREGNANT/NURSING MOTHERS, INFANTS, AND YOUNG CHILDREN

The opportunity to use pure, natural essential oils for your young family is such a blessing and will add so many tools to your parenting tool box. How I have wished that I had my oils when my children were small!

The recommendations for using essential oils are broad, and the information available can be confusing to those just starting out. Much of the information is based upon using poor quality essential oils, as was mentioned previously in this book. I recommend you seek out credible sources, do your own research, and find your own level of comfort for this season in your life. Young Living essential oils are SO much safer than many other common products to which most children are exposed every day! Every mother wants to use the best and safest products for her family, and Young Living offers many wonderful options, including specific product lines for babies and children. Check out the Suggested Resources section at the end of this book for some books to help guide you in your oily journey.

Many of the creations in this book may be used on children. If you are in doubt, start by applying a small amount on your child. You may also choose to further dilute before using on your little ones.

## CARING FOR YOUR OILS

Essential oils are chemically complex. The chemical compounds in them are best protected when they are kept away from light, air and extreme heat. Treat them carefully and avoid leaving them inside a hot car in the summertime. If your oils are accidentally exposed to heat, take them where it is cool and let them return to normal temperature without removing the lids. In my experience, undiluted oils have no shelf life, meaning they never expire. Some Young Living blends are pre-diluted. These oils may eventually expire due to the vegetable-based carrier oil they contain. However, because the essential oils will preserve the fatty oils, even the blends will remain good for a long time.

## STORING YOUR OILY CREATIONS

I always recommend glass, ceramic, or stainless steel for storing your DIY projects. This is especially important with citrus oils. Because light can cause oxidation of essential oils, the best choice of containers is dark-colored, glass bottles. If you use clear glass, be aware that over time you may need to add more essential oils to your creation. I only recommend using plastic bottles for spray cleaner bottles (heavily diluted) and for soap pump dispensers. Store your creations in a drawer, cabinet, or other place away from direct light.

# Recipes

Now for the very best part…let's start creating. Imagine me in my country kitchen with my apron on and my kitchen counters covered with supplies. That's how I roll. Go big or go home! I would rather tackle ten recipes in one day and have all the homemade creations needed to last my family for six months than to make recipes one at a time. I have been experimenting with recipes for more than three years, and these are my keepers. I hope you love them like I do.

# Pampering

## LOTION BARS

Create your own natural lotion in a convenient, non-messy bar.

- 1.8 oz. cocoa butter
- 1.0 oz. Shea butter
- 2.0 oz. beeswax pellets
- 1 tsp. vitamin E oil
- 2 oz. coconut oil
- 10 drops Orange essential oil
- 6 drops Geranium essential oil

Place a small glass bowl or jar inside a shallow pot. Add enough water to cover about 1/3 of the jar. Add all the ingredients except for essential oils to glass jar and bring surrounding water to a gentle boil. When the ingredients in the jar are melted, turn stove off and carefully remove the jar from the pot. Add essential oils and pour into soap molds. When bars are cool, they will pop right out of the molds. If you are gifting these, it's best to keep them refrigerated, especially if your home is a bit warm.

## PERFUME SPRITZER

- 2 Tbsp. olive oil or other carrier oil
- 30-40 total drops essential oils, choose from the combos listed below
- 2 Tbsp. distilled water
- Glass storage jar
- Perfume spritzer bottle

Mix olive oil and essential oils in jar, and shake gently for about 30 seconds. Allow the mixture to rest for 4-6 weeks. Add distilled water and shake again for several minutes before pouring into spritzer bottle. Shake gently prior to using.

**My combos:**

> **Perfect Peace:** 8 drops White Angelica™, 15 drops Lavender, 10 drops Bergamot
>
> **Fresh n Free:** 10 drops Peppermint, 15 drops Patchouli, 12 drops Lavender
>
> **Radiant Blooms:** 6 drops Geranium, 15 drops Ylang Ylang, 12 drops Lemon Myrtle

## PERFUME SOLID

1 Tbsp. beeswax crystals or pellets

1 Tbsp. almond oil

Essential oils, choose from one of the blends below (or create your own)

Small glass jars

Melt beeswax over a double boiler. Once the beeswax has melted, stir in almond oil. Remove from heat and allow to cool. Add essential oils and transfer mixture to storage jars to harden. (See the "Just for Him" section for a cologne solid.)

**Suggested Blends:**

> **Sweet Whisper:** 15 drops White Angelica™ & 10 drops Lavender
>
> **Happy Meadows:** 5 drops Geranium & 10 drops Orange

## BATH SALTS

1 cup Epsom salt

6-7 total drops of your favorite essential oils (or choose from suggestions below)

8 oz. glass jar

Combine bath salts and essential oils. Pour 1/2 cup salts in the bottom of empty bathtub, and fill with warm water. Soak for up to 30 minutes. You may gradually increase to up to 1 cup of bath salts per bath. Epsom salts can lower your blood pressure and bath salts can be rather detoxifying. Start slowly, drinking plenty of water before, during, and after bathing, and rise slowly as you get out of the tub. If you are taking blood pressure medication, use extra caution.

**Essential Oil Combinations:**
  **Muscle Relaxing:** Peppermint, Wintergreen
  **Runner's Salts:** Lemongrass and Copaiba
  **Sleepytime:** Lavender, Cedarwood
  **Uplifting:** Lemon, Peppermint
  **Detoxing:** Lemon, Purification®
  **Stress Relief:** Stress Away™, Frankincense
  **Feeling Romantic:** Ylang Ylang, Sensation™, Shutran™, Joy™

## BODY BUTTER/LOTION

This is a versatile base for many different creams. It can be used as a moisturizing foot cream (add oils for supporting circulation and skin), a soothing baby lotion, (try Gentle Baby™ or Lavender essential oil), or other lotion or cream.

  1/2 cup extra-virgin olive oil
  1/2 cup coconut oil
  1/2 cup distilled water
  2 oz. beeswax pellets
  1 Tbsp. vitamin E oil
  20-30 total drops essential oil (my favorites are Lavender,
    Cedarwood, Orange, Lime, Lemon, Peppermint)
  Glass jars

Place olive oil, coconut oil, water, and beeswax pellets over a double boiler. Warm mixture on low, heating just enough to melt the ingredients, stirring frequently until ingredients are blended and melted. As soon as the ingredients are blended, pour into a mixing bowl and beat with an electric mixer. When slightly cool to the touch, add the vitamin E oil and selected essential oils. Beat for another few minutes and refrigerate for 5 minutes. Remove from refrigerator and beat on medium speed for another 3-4 minutes. The body butter should be congealed, smooth, and creamy. If it's still too warm and liquefied, you may need to repeat refrigerating and blending until completely cooled and smooth. The goal is to prevent separation or lumps by mixing the body butter as it cools. Once fully blended, transfer to desired jars.

## CUTICLE/NAIL OIL
   1 Tbsp. vitamin E oil
   1 Tbsp. almond Oil
   5 drops Geranium or Tea Tree essential oil
   5 drops Lavender essential oil
   3 drops Lemon essential oil
   Dark glass dropper bottle

Mix together and place in small dark glass dropper bottle. Apply to nail cuticles and massage.

## FOAMING FACE WASH
   1 oz. castile soap (preferably unscented)
   Essential oils, choose from combinations below
   Foaming hand soap container

Add castile soap to an empty foaming hand soap dispenser. Add essential oils from the choices below. Top off with distilled water until bottle is 3/4 full.

### Essential oil combination for normal skin:
   2 drops Frankincense
   3 drops Geranium
   4 drops Orange
   2 drops Lavender

**Essential oil combination for acne prone skin (great for teens!):**
2 drops Frankincense
3 drops Purification®
3 drops Lemon
4 drops Tea Tree
2 drops Lavender

## LUSCIOUS LASHES

Add one drop each of Cedarwood, Frankincense, and Lavender essential oil to your tube of mascara. Enjoy healthy, long lashes and the pleasant aroma!

## ROMANCE MASSAGE OIL

3 oz. carrier oil of your choice (grapeseed, extra-virgin olive oil, almond oil, or YL V-6™)
8-10 drops essential oils, choose from combinations listed below
5 oz. glass jar

Mix carrier oil and selected essential oils. Gently blend as needed. Store in a glass jar.

**Suggested EO Combinations:**
Stress Away™ and Peppermint*
Lavender and Peppermint*
Ylang Ylang
Sensation™
Shutran™
Coriander and Goldenrod
Coriander and Peppermint*
*Optional: for a warming effect, add a drop of Black Pepper essential oil in place of Peppermint.*

# Sugar Scrubs

We don't pamper ourselves enough! Sugar scrubs make fabulous gifts for both men and women. Small jelly jars are the perfect size for scrubs. Keep in mind that some people prefer them with an oilier consistency, while others like them drier. You can adjust the consistency by adding a bit more oil or sugar. There is no wrong answer, and I promise you can't mess them up.

*Note: Sugar is not great for our bodies, especially when we consume it. When we use sugar on our skin, it will absorb into our skin to some degree. Most people do not use sugar scrubs daily but as an occasional spa pampering treatment. I do not recommend using these on your face. Instead, choose from the fabulous Young Living skin care products that are more suited for the delicate skin of your face. One of my favorites is the Satin Facial Scrub™. If you prefer to avoid using sugar on your skin, you can still use these recipes and alter them by using sea salt, oatmeal, coffee grounds and/or ground frankincense resin in place of the sugar.*

## LEMON SUGAR DETOX SCRUB

Lemon sugar scrub was one of the first recipes that I tried. It works amazingly and lasts for a long time. I use this in the shower for shaving, and it is great in the winter when hands and feet get dry. Lemon is also very detoxifying and is great for the skin! Because this contains Lemon essential oil, it should be stored in a glass jar. If you use a clear jar, you may need to add more essential oil over time.

1 cup granulated sugar
1/3 - 1/2 cup grapeseed oil
Juice from 1/4 lemon
20 drops Lemon essential oil
Glass jars

Mix in glass bowl until well blended and place in jars.

## FALL SUGAR SCRUB

1 cup brown sugar
1/2 cup olive oil
2-3 Tbsp. honey
1 Tbsp. vanilla extract
5 drops Cinnamon bark essential oil
5 drops Clove essential oil
3 drops Thieves® essential oil
*Optional: 3-5 drops Orange essential oil*
Glass jars

Mix in glass bowl until well blended and place in jars.

## ORANGE CREAMSICLE SUGAR SCRUB

1 cup coconut oil
1 cup sugar
1 tsp. vitamin E oil
1 tsp. vanilla extract
15 drops Orange essential oil
10 drops Stress Away™ essential oil
Glass jars

Mix in glass bowl until well blended and place in jars.

## JAVA ORANGE SUGAR SCRUB

1/2 cup brown sugar
1/4 cup coconut oil
1/4 cup coffee grounds
5 drops Orange essential oil
2 drops Clove essential oil
3 drops Thieves® essential oil
2 drops Ginger essential oil
2 drops Cinnamon bark essential oil
Glass jars

Mix in glass bowl until well blended and place in jars. Apply to feet with a scrubby. Rinse.

# Self-Care Products

## WATERLESS HAND CLEANER

Think cars, purses, and back packs! No sink or soap, no problem!
Port-a-potty relief! Clean hands on the go!

Aloe vera juice
10 drops Thieves® essential oil
1 Tbsp. vitamin E oil
Distilled water
2 oz. dark glass bottle

Fill container 2/3 full of aloe vera. Add Thieves®, vitamin E oil,
and top off with water. Give it a good shake and add a label.

## LIQUID HAND SOAP

1 oz. castile soap
1 Tbsp. vitamin E oil
Selected essential oils (for a total of about 10-15 drops)
Distilled water

Foaming hand soap container (recycled or purchased new)
In an empty, clean hand soap pump, add castile soap, vitamin E
oil, and selected essential oils. Some of my favorite combos are
Peppermint/Lemon, Spearmint/Lemon, Orange/Peppermint,
Spearmint/Tea Tree/Lemon, Lavender/Orange, and Tangerine/
Lemon. Add water until pump is 3/4 full and replace top. Gently
tip and allow a few minutes for ingredients to combine.

## HAIR CONDITIONER/RINSE

Hair conditioners tend to build up on hair. This rinse gives your hair a break and leaves it clean, soft, and tangle-free. The essential oils in the recipe conceal the ACV smell. I suggest using this in place of conditioner every other hair wash.

1/4 cup Bragg's® apple cider vinegar (ACV)
5 drops each Lavender, Cedarwood, Tea Tree essential oil
9 oz. distilled water

To an old shampoo bottle (recycle!), add Bragg's® ACV. Next add essential oils and distilled water. Generously coat your hair as soon as you get in the shower and allow to soak in while you shower or bathe. Rinse just before hopping out! Works great!

## BODY WASH

1/2 cup coconut milk
2/3 cup Dr. Bronner's® castile soap
1 Tbsp. vitamin E oil
5 drops of Tea Tree essential oil
3 drops Peppermint essential oil
1 Tbsp. vegetable glycerin

Combine all ingredients in a bottle. An old shampoo bottle with squeeze top works great.

## LEAVE-IN CONDITIONING TREATMENT

This conditioning treatment soaks into hair overnight. It leaves hair healthy and moisturized. Be prepared to wash your hair 3-4 times the following day. I recommend using this treatment monthly for normal hair, and more for excessively dry or damaged hair.

2 oz. castor oil
10 drops Tea Tree essential oil
6 drops Rosemary essential oil

8 drops Cedarwood essential oil
2 oz. dark glass bottle

Mix ingredients together in bottle. Massage 1-2 Tbsp. into hair and leave in 20 minutes or overnight. Rinse and shampoo thoroughly.

## CONDITIONING SPRAY FOR HAIR
8 drops Tea Tree essential oil
6 drops Lavender essential oil
6 drops Cedarwood essential oil
6 drops Bergamot essential oil
1-2 drops of jojoba oil
Distilled water
3 oz. glass spray bottle

Combine all ingredients in spray bottle. Add distilled water to fill bottle.

Shake thoroughly before each use. Spray on damp, clean hair for nourishment and amazing aromatherapy benefits!

## DEODORANT
If you are using a commercial deodorant, I MUST emphasize how critically important it is for you to make a change. Conventional deodorants contain aluminum, which is a toxic metal. It is nearly impossible for our bodies to get rid of aluminum or other metals on their own, so these toxins get stored away in our tissues. Our bodies are made to release toxins through our skin, particularly our armpits. By "blocking" the pores of our armpits with conventional deodorants, we are essentially keeping the toxins in. Deodorants also contain other harmful chemicals, including artificial fragrances and petroleum, that are best avoided as well. You can make the switch to a natural deodorant. You may need to try a few recipes to find one that works well for you, but it will be

100% worth the effort. For health's sake, this should be one of the very first changes you make.

*Note: Often when switching to a natural deodorant, your armpits will detox. This is temporary, and after consistent use you will eventually experience less body odor. In the beginning, you may need to reapply during the day, especially when exercising or if you are outside in the heat all day. Also keep in mind that each person has a unique body chemistry. I have provided a couple different recipes so that you may find the one that works best for you.*

## CREAM DEODORANT

The recipe is my personal favorite to use year-round. I have tried both of the recipes listed here (and many others) but this is the one to which I continually return. You will gradually get used to applying your deodorant with your fingers.

   1/4 cup aluminum-free baking soda
   1/4 cup arrowroot powder or cornstarch
   6-8 Tbsp. coconut oil
   10 drops Purification® essential oil
   Small glass jars

Combine baking soda and arrowroot powder or cornstarch. Gradually add coconut oil and work it in with a spoon until it maintains a firm but pliable texture. If it is too wet, add a bit more arrowroot powder or cornstarch to thicken. Add essential oil and store in glass jar.

## SOLID DEODORANT

2 Tbsp. beeswax pellets
2 Tbsp. Shea butter
2 Tbsp. coconut oil
2 1/2 Tbsp. arrowroot powder
1-2 Tbsp. glycerin
8-10 drops Purification® essential oil
8-10 drops Lavender or Tea Tree essential oil
Deodorant dispensers (recycled or new)

Combine all ingredients, except for essential oils, and melt using double boiler method. When melted, remove from heat and allow to cool. Add essential oils and pour into empty deodorant molds.

## NIGHTTIME FACE CREAM

These moisturizing creams are best stored in a cool, dark place, such as a bathroom drawer.

1/2 cup sunflower, grapeseed, or jojoba oil
Essential oils (options below)
6-8 oz. glass jar with lid, preferably dark-colored

### For Her:

10 drops Frankincense essential oil
8 drops Geranium essential oil
5 drops Lavender essential oil
4 drops Cedarwood essential oil
5 drops Tea Tree essential oil, optional, for acne prone skin

### For Him:

5 drops Idaho Blue Spruce essential oil
4 drops Tea Tree essential oil
6 drops Cedarwood essential oil
3 drops Frankincense essential oil

Combine all ingredients and place in jar. Apply to clean skin as needed.

## LIP BALM

- 2 Tbsp. cocoa butter
- 2 Tbsp. coconut oil
- 2 Tbsp. grapeseed oil
- 2 Tbsp. beeswax pellets
- 5 drops essential oil (such as Grapefruit, Lavender, Orange or Peppermint)
- 1/4 tsp. vitamin E oil
- Lip balm tubes or containers

Combine cocoa butter, coconut oil, grapeseed oil, and beeswax pellets in a glass canning jar. Fill a pot 1/3 with water. Create a double boiler by placing the canning jar in the pot. Bring water to a gentle boil over medium heat. Stir constantly until all ingredients melt and form a uniform mixture. Remove from heat and carefully remove the jar from the pot. (Alternatively, you can use a handy dip-sized crockpot to melt the fatty oils.) Allow the mixture to cool for 1-2 minutes, and stir in essential oils and vitamin E oil. Carefully pour mixture into 4-6 small glass or plastic lip balm containers or jars. (I love to use pipettes to fill the lip balm tubes!) Allow the lip balm to cool and harden completely before use.

## BEAUTY EYE CREAM

- 1 Tbsp. coconut oil
- 1 Tbsp. Shea butter
- 2 drops each of Frankincense, Lavender, Geranium and Lemon, and Sandalwood essential oil
- Small glass jar

Using double boiler method, melt all ingredients and pour into a small glass jar. Apply around eyes morning and night.

## HOMEMADE MOUTHWASH

4 oz. distilled water

1/2 tsp. high quality sea salt

4 drops Clove essential oil

4 drops Rosemary essential oil

4 drops Peppermint essential oil

4 drops Lemon essential oil

4-6 oz. glass jar

Add sea salt to glass jar or bottle. Then add essential oils. Allow oils to soak into salt a bit and add the distilled water. Shake well before each use.

# Household Cleaning

## SCRUBBY SURFACE CLEANER

This cleaner is great for cleaning countertops, sinks, tile, and showers.

6-8 oz. baking soda (about half a jar)
6-8 oz. washing soda (about half a jar)
1 capful Thieves® Household Cleaner
10 drops Lemon essential oil
16 oz. glass jar

Mix together in a glass or stainless steel bowl. Pour mixture into glass jar.

## DAILY SHOWER SPRAYS

Research has revealed that a vent over your shower that leads to the outside of your house is necessary to keep fungi from growing in your bathroom. For extra protection, keep your shower or bathtub fresh and clean without scrubbing. Spray one of these mixtures on shower surfaces daily after showering. No need to rinse.

### SHOWER CLEANER #1

1/2 cup vinegar
20 drops Lemon essential oil
Distilled water
22 oz. spray bottle

Combine vinegar and lemon essential oil in spray bottle. Add distilled water to fill bottle.

## SHOWER CLEANER #2

1/3 cup vinegar
3 Tbsp. witch hazel
30 drops Lemon essential oil
3 Tbsp. castile soap
3 Tbsp. Thieves® Household Cleaner
24 oz. distilled water
24-32 oz. spray bottle

Mix all ingredients together and pour into spray bottle.

## SPARKLING TOILET

1 tsp. Thieves® Household Cleaner
1/4 cup baking soda
3-4 drops Lemon essential oil, optional

Thieves® Household Cleaner (THC) concentrate makes a wonderful toilet bowl cleaner. Use 1 part THC diluted with 30 parts water to clean outer surfaces, lid, and seat of commode. For inside the toilet bowl, combine THC and baking soda to make a paste. Clean with a sponge or scrub brush. For tougher toilet stains, simply add 3-4 drops of Lemon essential oil to the toilet water. Allow to sit overnight before flushing.

## GLASS CLEANER HACK

2 microfiber cloths
Water

Dampen one microfiber cloth and use to clean glass surfaces using circular motions. Dry with other cloth. This works like a charm on windows and mirrors and is completely chemical-free!

## LAUNDRY SOAP

1 cup baking soda
1 cup citric acid
2 cups washing soda
1/2 cup coarse sea salt
2 bars Dr. Bronner's® castile soap or pure glycerin soap
25 drops Lemon essential oil
Large canning jars or recycled glass jars

Grate bars of castile soap by hand or in a food processor. Add remaining ingredients. Stir and place in glass jar. Use 1 tablespoon for an average load or 2 tablespoons for an extra-large or particularly soiled load.

## LAUNDRY SPOT REMOVER

3 Tbsp. hydrogen peroxide
3 Tbsp. washing soda
6 Tbsp. water
2 drops Lemon essential oil
2-4 oz. glass jar

Combine ingredients in glass jar. Rub into stains and wash as usual.

## LAUNDRY SPOT REMOVER #2

4 Tbsp. Thieves® Dish Soap
10 drops Lemon essential oil
Small squeeze bottle

Combine ingredients and pour into squeeze container Apply to stains using a toothbrush.

*Tip: Thieves® Dish Soap also works well as a spot remover. Simply apply a dab of dish soap to the spot and launder as usual.*

## ALL-PURPOSE CLEANER

1 Tbsp. witch hazel
3 drops Tea Tree essential oil
3 drops Peppermint essential oil
3 drops Lemon essential oil
4 oz. distilled water
Small spray bottle

Combine all ingredients in spray bottle. Shake before using. Spray surfaces well, allow to sit for a few minutes, and wipe clean.

## ALL-PURPOSE CLEANER #2

4 oz. liquid castile soap
10 drops Lemon essential oil
10 drops Thieves® essential oil
24 oz. distilled water
Large spray bottle

Combine all ingredients in spray bottle. Shake before using. Spray surfaces well, allow to sit for a few minutes, and wipe clean.

## HOUSEHOLD CLEANER WIPES

1 Tbsp. aloe vera juice
1 Tbsp. castile soap, unscented
1 Tbsp. vitamin E oil
1 tsp. olive oil
15 drops Thieves® essential oil
2 cups distilled water
Roll of sturdy, high quality paper towels *(preferably unbleached)*
Cylindrical Rubbermaid® container

Mix together aloe vera, castile soap, vitamin E oil, olive oil and essential oil. Stir in distilled water. Cut entire roll of paper towels in half using a serrated knife. Place cut roll inside cylindrical container. Gently pour soap mixture over paper towels. Shake a few times to distribute. After the mixture soaks in, you should be able to remove the cardboard center.

## CARPET FRESHENER

This is a great remedy for the "aroma" our furry family members leave behind!

Baking soda
Glass pizza cheese shaker (or a mason jar with holes punched in the lid)
Essential oils for air freshening (Purification®, Lemon, Orange, Citrus Fresh™)

Fill bottle with baking soda and add 25-35 drops of essential oils. Shake on carpet before vacuuming.

## WOOD RESTORE

1 oz. Thieves® Household Cleaner
20 drops Citrus Fresh™ or Orange essential oil
1 cup olive oil
Small dark glass bottle

Mix ingredients together and apply to wood surfaces with a microfiber cloth. Allow mixture to soak into wood overnight. If needed, rub gently with a clean, dry microfiber cloth to remove excess oils.

# Health & Wellness

## CHEST RUB

1/2 cup coconut oil
1/2 cup Shea butter
1/3 cup almond oil
1 Tbsp. vitamin E oil
10 drops each Peppermint, Eucalyptus Radiata, Wintergreen
and Ravintsara essential oils
Large glass jar

Melt coconut oil, Shea butter, and almond oil in a double boiler. When thoroughly melted, cool to room temperature and add vitamin E oil and essential oils. Pour into glass container. Apply to chest to support the respiratory system.

## AFTER-SUN RUB

Aloe vera juice (no additives)
5 drops Peppermint essential oil
10 drops Lavender essential oil
1 Tbsp. vitamin E oil
2 oz. dark glass bottle

Fill bottle 3/4 full of aloe vera. Add remaining ingredients and a bit of distilled water. Shake and apply to sun-hot skin.

## BOO-BOO SPRAY

1/2 tsp. salt
5 drops Lavender essential oil
3 drops Purification® essential oil
3 drops Tea Tree essential oil
2 drops Dorado Azul™ essential oil
8 oz. distilled water
Dark-colored glass spray bottle

Combine essential oils and salt. Add water and shake. This can be sprayed on minor cuts and abrasions.

## NASAL IRRIGATION

3 drops Rosemary essential oil
3 drops Tea Tree essential oil
2 tsp. sea salt
Distilled water
Small glass jar

Add essential oils to salt and store in a glass jar. For nasal irrigation, add 1-teaspoon salt/EO mixture to distilled water and irrigate. Use as needed for support of sinus health.

## FRESH BREATH SPRAY

3 oz. distilled water
5 drops Peppermint essential oil
3 drops Lemon essential oil
4 drops Thieves® essential oil
3 oz. glass spray bottle

Combine all ingredients in spray bottle. Shake before using.

## SLEEPYTIME BALM

1/2 cup coconut oil
25 drops Lavender essential oil
25 drops Cedarwood essential oil
15 drops Sandalwood essential oil
4-6 oz. glass jar

Stir together coconut oil and essential oils and place in glass jar.
Apply to feet and/or chest at bedtime.

## SLEEPYTIME ROLLER BLEND

Extra-virgin olive oil or other carrier oil
15 drops Lavender essential oil
15 drops Cedarwood essential oil
10 drops Sandalwood essential oil
15 mL empty essential oil bottle (recycle!)
Stainless steel roller top

Fill empty 15 mL bottle halfway with carrier oil and add
essential oils. Apply stainless steel roller top. Roll on temples
or feet as needed.

## SPRINGTIME ROLLER BLEND

Carrier oil such as olive oil or almond oil
12 drops each Lavender, Lemon and Peppermint essential oils
15 mL empty essential oil bottle (recycle!)

Fill roller bottle halfway with carrier oil and add essential oils.
Apply roller top to bottle and roll on forehead, temples and/or
chest as needed. Be careful to keep oils away from eyes!

## HAPPY ME ROLLER BLEND

 Extra-virgin olive oil or other carrier oil
 15 drops Joy™ essential oil
 12 drops Orange essential oil
 10 drops Lemon essential oil
 15 mL empty essential oil bottle (recycle!)

Fill roller bottle halfway with carrier oil and add essential oils. Apply roller top to bottle and roll on forehead, temples, and/or chest as needed. Be sure to keep oils out of your eyes!

## BUG-OFF SPRAY

Since we live outside the city limits, this is a regular in our home. Put it to the test…you'll be impressed! It can also be used on your four-legged friends. Spray onto your hands and pet them, being careful to avoid your pet's face.

 1 Tbsp. witch hazel
 5 drops Thieves® essential oil
 5 drops Purification® essential oil
 5 drops Peppermint essential oil
 5 drops Citronella essential oil
 5 drops Lemongrass essential oil *(optional, for an extra boost)*
 Distilled water
 3 oz. Glass spray bottle

Mix witch hazel and essential oils together in glass spray bottle. Add water to fill bottle. Apply to skin and clothing as needed.

*Diffuser Tip: This is also a great combo for the diffuser when sitting outside! Use 2 drops each of the listed essential oils and camp out around the diffuser!*

# For the Little Ones

## BABY BOTTOM WIPES

1 Tbsp. aloe vera juice
1 Tbsp. castile soap, unscented
1 Tbsp. vitamin E oil
1 tsp. olive oil
5 drops Lavender essential oil
5 drops Tea Tree essential oil
2 cups distilled water
Roll of sturdy, high quality paper towels *(preferably unbleached)*
Cylindrical Rubbermaid® container

Mix together aloe vera, castile soap, vitamin E oil, olive oil, and essential oils. Stir in distilled water. Cut entire roll of paper towels in half using a serrated knife. Place cut roll inside cylindrical container. Carefully pour soap mixture over paper towels. Shake a few times to distribute. After the mixture soaks in, you should be able to remove the cardboard center.

## BOO-BOO SALVE

1/4 cup coconut oil
1/4 cup olive oil
1 Tbsp. beeswax pellets
10 drops Lavender essential oil
10 drops Lemon essential oil
10 drops Frankincense essential oil
5 drops Myrrh or Helichrysum essential oil
1 drop Peppermint essential oil
5 drops Tea Tree oil
Small jars or lip balm tubes

Melt coconut oil, olive oil, and beeswax in a double boiler. Cool slightly and add essential oils. Carefully pour into glass containers, jars, or lip balm tubes. Allow to harden before using. Apply to minor cuts and scrapes.

## BABY BOTTOM CREAM

1/4 cup coconut oil
1/4 cup olive oil
1 Tbsp. beeswax pellets
20 drops Gentle Baby™ essential oil
5 drops Lavender essential oil
Small jars or lip balm tubes

Melt coconut oil, olive oil, and beeswax in a double boiler. Cool slightly and add essential oils. Carefully pour into glass containers, jars, or lip balm tubes. Allow to harden before using.

## BUBBLE BATH

1 cup castile soap
2/3 cup liquid glycerin
5 drops Lavender essential oil
1/4 cup distilled water
Glass bottles or jar

Mix together castile soap, glycerin, and essential oil. Add water. Add 2 tablespoons to warm bath. *(Note: Use bubble bath with caution with little girls! If they tend to be prone to urinary tract infections, then bubble baths are a no-no. This recipe is made with the purest ingredients, so you may not find it to be a problem!)*

## PLAY DOUGH

2 cups flour
1 cup salt
2 cups water
1 Tbsp. vegetable oil
2 tsp. cream of tartar
Desired essential oils for aroma (try Orange, Peppermint, Lavender, Lime, Lemon, etc.)

Combine flour, salt, water, vegetable oil, and cream of tarter in a pot. Cook slowly over low heat until blended and no longer sticky. Remove from heat and add a few drops of desired essential oil. Store in an airtight container or zipper bag.

## SCENTED SENSORY RICE MIX

Add a few drops of your choice of essential oil to a zipper bag of rice. Use as a sensory activity for kiddos during winter or hot summer months. Place a plastic tablecloth on the kitchen floor and give them measuring cups, spoons, and scoops. So fun!

**Suggested essential oils:** Lavender, Orange, Lemon, Tangerine.

# Just for Him

## ROBUST LOTION

1/2 cup extra-virgin olive oil
1/2 cup coconut oil
1/2 cup water
2 oz. beeswax pellets
1 Tbsp. vitamin E oil
10 drops Idaho Blue Spruce essential oil
25 drops Peppermint essential oil
20 drops Mister™ essential oil
Glass jars

Place olive oil, coconut oil, water, and beeswax pellets over a double boiler. Heat mixture on low, heating just enough to melt the ingredients, stirring frequently until ingredients are blended and melted. As soon as the ingredients are blended, pour into a mixing bowl and beat with an electric mixer. When slightly cool to the touch, add the vitamin E oil and selected essential oils. Beat for another few minutes and refrigerate for 5 minutes. Remove from refrigerator and beat on medium speed for another 3-4 minutes. The lotion should be congealed, smooth, and creamy. If it's still too warm and liquefied, you may need to refrigerate and blend again until completely cooled and smooth. The goal is to prevent separation or lumps by mixing the body butter as it cools. Once fully blended, transfer to desired jars.

## COLOGNE SOLID

1 Tbsp. beeswax crystals or pellets
1 Tbsp. almond oil
Essential oils, choose from blends below (or create your own):
Small glass jars

Melt beeswax over a double boiler. Once the beeswax has melted, stir in almond oil. Remove from heat and allow to cool slightly. Add essential oils and transfer mixture to storage jars to harden.

**Every Man:** 15 drops Peppermint & 10 drops Cedarwood
**Man Up:** 15 drops Mister™ & 10 drops Peppermint
**To the Nines:** 20 drops Shutran™, 10 drops Cedarwood &
    5 drops Idaho Blue Spruce

## WORKING MAN'S HAND SCRUB

3/4 cup Epsom salt
1-2 Tbsp. Thieves® Household Cleaner
2 Tbsp. castile soap (I like Dr. Bronner's®)
1/4 cup coconut oil
8 oz. glass jar

Stir together and store in glass jar. Use about a tablespoon to clean hands.

## BEARD OIL

1 oz. jojoba oil
1 Tbsp. vitamin E oil
10 drops Mister™ essential oil
4 drops Tea Tree essential oil
3 drops Lavender essential oil
1 drop Peppermint essential oil
Small dark glass jar

Blend all ingredients. Store in a dark glass jar and apply as needed to soften facial hair.

## DATE NIGHT COLOGNE
1 oz. witch hazel
1 oz. distilled water
7-8 drops Shutran™ essential oil
3 drops Idaho Blue Spruce essential oil
1-2 drops Northern Lights Black Spruce essential oil
1-2 drops Orange essential oil
2-3 oz. dark-colored spray bottle.

Combine all ingredients in spray bottle. Apply liberally and prepare for a happy wife.

## CAMOUFLAGE WOODS BLEND
1 oz. grapeseed oil
5 drops Cedarwood essential oil
5 drops Pine essential oil
3 drops Idaho Blue Spruce essential oil
4 drops Idaho Balsam Fir essential oil
Small glass jar

Mix in jar and apply before hunting. To make a spray, omit grapeseed oil and add to 3 oz. spray bottle with a tablespoon of vodka or witch hazel and distilled water.

## STINKY SHOE POWDER
1/4 cup baking soda
10-20 drops Purification® essential oil
Glass pizza-shaker bottle (or a mason jar with holes punched in the lid)

Combine in shaker bottle and sprinkle into shoes. Allow to sit overnight, and pour out excess before wearing shoes.

## GYM GUY/SPORTS BLEND

1/2 cup coconut oil
10 drops Peppermint essential oil
10 drops Copaiba essential oil
10 drops Lemongrass essential oil
10 drops Wintergreen essential oil
15 drops PanAway® essential oil
5 drops Frankincense essential oil
Small glass jar

Blend coconut oil and essential oils in a glass bowl and place in small jars. Best if stored away from light. Massage into sore or stressed areas. Also works to encourage circulation before exercise.

# Miscellaneous

## SWEET DREAMS SPRAY

15 drops Dream Catcher™ essential oil
5 drops Lavender essential oil
Distilled water
3 oz. spray bottle

Mix all ingredients in spray bottle and lightly mist pillows at bedtime.

## VEGGIE WASH

1/3 cup apple cider vinegar (Braggs® is my favorite)
2 cups distilled water
15 drops Lemon essential oil
5 drops Orange essential oil
Dark glass bottle

Mix all ingredients together and store in dark glass jar or bottle. Add 3 tablespoons to a bowl of water. Soak produce for 5 minutes. Rinse.

## VEGGIE SPRAY

This is great for taking on-the-go! Carry in a purse or backpack for traveling. Follow Veggie Wash recipe above and pour into a spray bottle. Spray on fruits and veggies, rub and rinse.

## DRYER BALLS

100% wool yarn skein – light colored (Available at most craft
stores. Be sure to get 100% wool.)
Piece of panty hose
Desired essential oils

Start a ball of yarn by tightly rolling yarn around fingers.
Continue rolling until it is about the size of a tennis ball. Tuck
loose end into the ball with the end of a paper clip. Place balls
into a length of panty hose and tie knots on both sides. Boil in
water on the stove for ten minutes. Place the balls (still inside
the panty hose) into the clothes washer on hot cycle and run
through wash. Next place the dryer balls (still inside the panty
hose) in clothes dryer. After a full cycle in the dryer, they should
be tightly woven and "felted". Felted yarn cannot be taken apart;
it is so tightly woven that it remains a tight ball forever. You can
now add desired essential oils and use in place of dryer sheets in
the dryer. Some essential oils that I love to add to my dryer balls
are Orange, Lemon, Lime, Tangerine, Purification®, Citrus Fresh™
and Lavender. These balls also decrease the dry time of your
laundry by separating the clothes nicely during drying.

*Gift giving tip: These make an inexpensive gift that people love to
receive! I often times pair them with a citrus oil like Citrus Fresh™
or Orange essential oil.*

## KITTY LITTER BOX DEODORIZER

4 cups baking soda
25 drops Purification® essential oil

Combine ingredients and sprinkle in bottom of pan before
litter is added. May also sprinkle another 1-2 tablespoons on
top of litter.

## BUG-OFF FOR FOUR-LEGGED FRIENDS

1 Tbsp. olive oil

1-2 drops each Purification®, Lavender, Lemon, and Geranium
essential oils

Mix together and apply to the back of the neck of the dog or cat.

## ROOM SPRAY/DEODORIZER

1 oz. witch hazel or rubbing alcohol

10 oz. distilled water

Total of 16 drops essential oils (choose from combos below)

12 oz. glass spray bottle

Mix witch hazel or alcohol and water together and pour into
spray bottle. Add desired essential oil combo.

**Suggested essential oil combos:**

Lavender/Peppermint, Lemon/Orange, Spearmint/Orange,
Thieves®/Lemon, Purification®/Lemon

## COOLING SPRAY/AFTER-SUN SPRAY

This is fantastic when your skin needs a little nourishment
after sun exposure or just to refresh during the heat of the day.
Especially refreshing when stored in refrigerator.

1 Tbsp. witch hazel

3 oz. distilled water

5 drops Lavender essential oil

8 drops Peppermint essential oil

6 oz. glass spray bottle

Mix witch hazel and water together and place in spray bottle. Add
essential oils.

# Bar Soap

My favorite way to make soap is the hot process method. Why? Remember that essential oils lose their therapeutic value and aroma when they are exposed to intense heat. During hot processing, the soap mixture is cooled before adding essential oils, which preserves the therapeutic properties and aroma of the oil and gives a better scent. With cold processing, this isn't possible because the saponification (cooking) takes place over time – while the soap is in the mold – and the oils must be added before they go into the mold. Therefore, hot processing yields soap with a better aroma and preserves the therapeutic benefits of the essential oils. The preservation of the therapeutic value of the oils is of utmost importance to me as it gives additional value and effectiveness to my soap.

**TIPS FOR SUCCESS:**

- Read through this entire chapter several times and gather all of your supplies before beginning.
- Avoid distractions. The few times I have created less-than-perfect soap, it was because I had distractions in my workspace.
- Lye soap is a combination of fatty

Figuring the amount of essential oil to use in soaps is a matter of preference and can take some trial and error. Typically, citrus oils and lighter-scented oils will require more essential oil to get the desired fragrance. Oils that have a stronger scent, such as Peppermint and Spearmint don't require as much. A larger batch of soap will obviously require more EO than a smaller one. As a general rule, I almost always use at least half of a 15 mL bottle (0.25 oz.). There's no wrong answer, so be sure to make notes and adjust to your personal preference.

oils, lye, and water in specific proportions based on the amount and type of fatty oils used. The lye/water solution is what causes heat (saponification) and turns the mixture into soap. The key to soap-making is to take a simple recipe and follow the directions exactly. If you are going to alter the recipes included here (or any other soap recipe), you must recalculate your lye and water ratio with a soap calculator. These are easy to find online or even as an app for your smartphone. As a beginner, you are better off following a tried-and-true recipe (like one of those included here) before venturing to create your own unique recipe.

**SAFETY TIPS FOR WORKING WITH LYE:**

- Always keep lye out of reach of children and pets.
- Keep all pets out of the room while making soap.
- Keep your soap-making supplies separate from your other kitchen utensils.
- Label specific utensils for use with lye, and don't use them for other purposes.
- Don't lean over the pot while mixing lye and water or while blending to avoid inhaling the fumes.
- Keep a bottle of vinegar on the counter when using lye. In case of accidental contact on skin, vinegar will neutralize the burn.

**ARE YOU READY? LET'S GET STARTED MAKING SOAP!**

## SOAP MAKING SUPPLY LIST

Most soap-making supplies are readily available from Amazon.

- Various fatty oils – coconut, palm, sweet almond, etc. (Check specific recipe.)
- 100% Lye (sodium hydroxide or NaOH) (found online or in drain cleaner section of hardware stores)
- Distilled water
- Kitchen scale that measures ounces
- Kitchen thermometer (I prefer digital or infrared)
- Immersion blender
- Crockpot, medium-large (preferably with low and medium settings and removable crock. Mine is tall, rather than oval, which is preferable to be able to fully submerse the blender.)
- Safety glasses
- Handkerchief or face mask
- Gloves, rubber or disposable
- Soap mold (If you don't want to purchase a soap mold, you can use small paper milk cartons, glass bread pans, or other suitable container(s). Almost anything may be used as a mold, as long as it isn't aluminum, tin, or copper.)
- Kitchen utensils specific for soap making (spoons, bowls, etc. – Do not use aluminum, tin or copper for soap making)
- Glass bowls – various sizes
- Shallow pan for cooling bath, such as pie pan
- Towels, kitchen size
- pH strips (specific to soap-making)
- Vinegar (for accidental lye on skin)

# BAR SOAP RECIPES

## NATURALLY NOURISHING SOAP
**Lye/Water**
    5.36 oz. lye (sodium hydroxide)
    12.5 oz. distilled Water
**Fatty oils**
    16 oz. coconut oil
    9 oz. olive oil
    8 oz. Shea Butter
    5 oz. grapeseed oil
    Desired essential oils and/or additives

## SIMPLY CLEAN SOAP
**Lye/Water**
    3.87 oz. lye (sodium hydroxide)
    9.24 oz. distilled Water
**Fatty oils**
    14 oz. coconut oil
    12 oz. grapeseed oil
    1 oz. jojoba oil
    1 oz. vitamin E oil
    Desired essential oils and/or additives

## ADDITIVES IN SOAP

Once you practice making soap, you may want to get a bit more creative with your recipes. Consider using oatmeal, coffee grounds, flower buds, or any other additives that you want to try. Like essential oils, the amount of additives to use is based on your personal preference. More additives will produce a more exfoliating bar. For a typical batch of soap, I use 1/4 - 1/2 cup of additives.

**Some of my favorite combos:**
Lavender EO & oatmeal
Northern Lights Black Spruce EO, Pine EO &
   Cinnamon Bark EO
Cinnamon Bark EO, Nutmeg EO, Clove EO & Coffee
Ylang Ylang EO & Peppermint EO
Lemongrass EO & Peppermint EO
Tea Tree EO & oatmeal

## PROCEDURE

1. Gather all tools and prepare your work area. A large, clean counter and stovetop is ideal.
2. Assemble your supplies: crockpot, several bowls, oven mitts, implements for measuring, stirring, etc., thermometer, kitchen scale, and soap mold. (If you aren't sure whether or not your container is aluminum, you can line it with freezer paper or waxed paper.) Prepare the molds with old kitchen towels underneath to catch spills.
3. Using a kitchen scale, weigh the solid fatty oils in the recipe. Melt in a crockpot or double boiler. Add liquid fatty oils to melted mixture.
4. Remove fatty oils from heat and allow to begin cooling.
5. Weigh distilled water in a glass bowl.
6. Before handling lye, PUT ON YOUR SAFETY GLASSES, GLOVES, AND A HANDKERCHIEF OVER YOUR MOUTH/NOSE. Weigh lye in a dry glass container that has been labeled for lye.
7. Slowly pour the measured lye granules into the distilled water. NEVER POUR WATER INTO LYE. ALWAYS POUR LYE INTO WATER. ("Snow on the lake" is a phrase to help your remember to add the lye to the water and never the other way around.) Stand back from the mixture so that you don't directly inhale resulting fumes. The mixture will be

cloudy at first, and as it naturally heats, it will turn clear. Stir constantly and gently, with a stainless steel spoon, until the mixture is clear and all lye granules are dissolved. Set aside.

8. Cool lye mixture to 120°F. To speed cooling, you may use a cool water bath if desired. (Place the lye mixture carefully inside a pie pan of cold water. Be sure that the cooling bath water doesn't overflow into the prepared lye mixture. Gently add a few handfuls of ice cubes to the water bath pan. Frequently test the temperature of the lye water until it is between 110°-120°F.)

9. Tip: Stir both lye mixture and oil mixture gently to cool. Both the fatty oil mixture and the lye mixture need to be within a range of 110°-120°F. If the oils cool too quickly, place them back on the stove or heat the crockpot briefly until they reach the ideal temperature. Turn crockpot off before continuing to the next step.

10. WHILE STILL WEARING SAFETY GLASSES AND GLOVES, slowly pour lye mixture into the oil mixture in crockpot. Stir briefly to mix the ingredients. Place immersion blender in the pot, making sure the blade is completely immersed in the mixture to avoid splatters.

11. Pulse the low button on the immersion blender. Just hold it firmly (use two hands if you feel unsteady). You do not need to lift the immersion blender; keep it completely immersed in the mixture while blending.

12. After about 5-10 minutes of blending, the mixture should be thickened and you should begin to see a cloudy appearance on the surface. This is called "trace". These recipes will somewhat resemble vanilla pudding in both color and consistency. When you remove the spoon or blender, you can still see a "trace" of it in the top of the soap. Stop blending when you see trace and your soap resembles this thick pudding consistency.

13. Turn crockpot on low and cook for 30 minutes to an hour. It will begin to look waxy and the top outer edges will dry out and begin to fold onto itself. The soap will no longer look like thick vanilla pudding on the edges, but will have a waxy/translucent look. When this occurs, stir well, replace crockpot lid and cook another 15 minutes.

14. The mixture above should be mostly translucent with some chunkiness to it. At this point, check the soap with a pH test strip. To do this, remove about 1/2-teaspoon of soap from crock with a spoon, add a bit of water to it to lather, it and place on the test strip. When pH measures between 7-10, your soap is done. Remove crock from base, and stir to cool mixture. (At this point, you no longer need protective wear.)

15. Check temperature regularly and add essential oils and additives, if desired, when soap reaches about 140-150°F. (If temperature gets much cooler than 140°F, it becomes too difficult to spread in the molds.) This is the magic of using hot process! By allowing your soap to cool a bit before adding essential oils, you are able to use much less EO and get a fabulous-smelling soap with all the therapeutic values of the essential oils.

16. Place soap into molds. You may remove as soon as soap has hardened enough to slide easily out of molds. I generally allow it to dry for several weeks, although it is safe to use immediately.

## FREQUENTLY ASKED QUESTIONS

1. **Is lye (sodium hydroxide) safe to be used in soap even though it is toxic in its raw form?**
Yes! Lye deserves to be handled with extreme caution, but after it is properly processed, it is completely nontoxic. Because of the chemical reaction that takes place during processing, there is actually no lye present in the finished product.

2. **Do you use lye soap faster or is it softer than conventional bar soaps?**

    Lye soap is a bit softer in my opinion. This somewhat depends on the oils and ratios that you use. Some ingredients will make a firmer soap. I have found that if I use all liquid fatty oils, the soap is too soft. Your soap will last longer if you keep it out of the water in the shower. Also, because they are so amazingly wonderful to use, we tend to use more of them to soap up!

3. **What type of additives are your favorites?**

    I have used lavender flower buds, dried chamomile buds, sugar, oatmeal, cinnamon, vanilla and essential oils.

4. **Which essential oils are your favorites for soap making?**

    I love them all, but I use Lemongrass the most. Lemongrass smells delicious and the aroma holds very well in soap. By now you know that I will only use Young Living essential oils for my family, but even with 100% pure therapeutic grade essential oils, some of the scent is lost during the soap-making process. Other essential oils that I love to use in soap are Peppermint, Spearmint, Christmas Spirit™, Orange, Tangerine, Stress Away™, Lavender, Lemon, Clove, Blue Spruce, Northern Lights Black Spruce and Ylang Ylang.

5. **Isn't it a bit expensive to use essential oils in your soap making?**

    I have calculated the cost of various soap recipes and it rarely comes to more than $15 for a batch that will last my family many months (not including essential oils). Once I add the essential oil, it generally costs about $25 per batch (depending on the oil I choose). It is well worth it in my opinion!

# Hosting DIY Classes

When I initially wrote this book, my goals were to provide a collection of my favorite recipes for personal use and for my oily family to use. After I wrote and published it, I realized that many of my friends were using my book to expand their business. DIY Classes are a great way to share your non-toxic lifestyle with friends and family and have some fun at the same time. People love to attend DIY classes and learn new things!

There are a few different ways that you can host your own DIY classes. My preference is a Themed Demo Class because it is less expensive for and requires less prep work by the hostess, making it much easier for others to duplicate. It also demonstrates how easy it is to create many DIY items and inspires attendees to go home and try some new recipes with their oils.

Unless you are charging for this event, limit your invites to members of your organization. Young Living is a business and your time is valuable. According to Young Living Policies and Procedures, sponsors are required to educate members of their team. Also, you may be limited to space in your home or business. Teaching about YL products at this event will also help grow your business through education and fun.

## THEMED DEMO CLASS

Choose a topic from this book (DIY for Kids, Spa Day, DIY Gift Giving, DIY Household Cleaning, DIY Roller Bottles, Soap Making, etc.). Advertise and invite friends to attend the free demo class. Select 3-5 recipes (unless it is a soap-making demo) from the book. During the class, demonstrate making the selected recipes in front of your guests. Do a door prize drawing and gift one or more of the items that you make to the winner(s). Provide recipes and ideas (or even a copy of this book) to your attendees.

## MAKE & TAKE

Decide on a theme or choose 3-5 simple recipes from this book to include in your class. Figure the cost of your expenses, and include the cost of the class in your invitation (typically around $5-$15). Advertise the class and require guests to RSVP by a specified date. This allows time for the hostess to gather needed supplies for all attendees. The hostess should provide all ingredients, jars or other containers, labels, and essential oils for the recipes. Attendees come and learn how to make several items and then take them home.

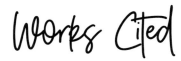

# Works Cited

Agency for Toxic Substances and Disease Registry. (2008, September). "Public Health Statement for Aluminum". Retrieved from: https://www.atsdr.cdc.gov/phs/phs.asp?id=1076&tid=34.

Bennett, James. (2013, August 3). "Petrolatum/Petroleum Jelly". *Cosmetics and Skin*. Retrieved from: http://cosmeticsandskin.com/bcb/petrolatum.php.

Cunningham, Vanessa. (2014, January 23). "10 Toxic Beauty Ingredients to Avoid". *Huffington Post*. Retrieved from: https://www.huffingtonpost.com/vanessa-cunningham/dangerous-beauty-products_b_4168587.html.

*Environmental Working Group*. (2018). Retrieved from: http://www.ewg.org.

Ettinger, Jill. (2015, February 20). "7 Ways to Avoid Parabens and Phthalates in Personal Care Products". *One Green Planet*. Retrieved from: http://www.onegreenplanet.org/lifestyle/how-to-avoid-parabens-and-phthalates-in-personal-care-products/.

Group, Edward. (2017, March 24). "New Research Indicates Aluminum in Deodorant Linked To Breast Cancer". *Global Healing Center*. Retrieved from: http://www.globalhealingcenter.com/natural-health/aluminum-and-breast-cancer.

Group, Edward. (2015, June 8). "Why You Should Use Aluminum-Free Deodorant". *Global Healing Center*. Retrieved from: https://www.globalhealingcenter.com/natural-health/why-you-should-use-aluminum-free-deodorant/.

Group, Edward. (2015, November 16). "Dangers of Fluoride". *Global Healing Center*. Retrieved from: https://www.globalhealingcenter.com/natural-health/how-safe-is-fluoride/.

James, Maia. (2013, January 14). "How to Avoid Pthalates (Even Though You Can't Avoid Pthalates)". *Huffington Post*. Retrieved from: https://www.huffingtonpost.com/maia-james/phthalates-health_b_2464248.html.

*Keeper of the Home*. (2012, April 24). "Eliminating Aluminum from Our Homes". Retrieved from: https://keeperofthehome.org/eliminating-aluminum-from-our-homes/.

*Medicine.net*. (2011, March 29). "Fluoride". Retrieved from: https://www.medicinenet.com/fluoride/supplements-vitamins.htm.

Mercola, Joseph. (2016, September 6). "Water Fluoridation Linked to

Diabetes and Low IQ". *Mercola.com.* Retrieved from: https://articles.
mercola.com/sites/articles/archive/2016/09/06/water-fluoridation-
diabetes-low-iq.aspx.

National Center for Biotechnology Information. (Accessed 2018, March 5).
*PubChem Compound Database.* Retrieved from: https://pubchem.ncbi.
nim.nih.gov/compound/1140.

Peltier, Karen. (2018, January 15). "Why You Should Avoid the Chemical
Additive Triclosan" *The Spruce.* Retrieved from: https://www.thespruce.
com/triclosan-how-its-used-avoid-it-1707033.

Ropp, Thomas. (2017, March 7). "The Dark Side of Propylene Glycol: Side
Effects and How to Avoid Them". *Honey Colony.* Retrieved from: https://
www.honeycolony.com/article/propylene-glycol/.

*Safer Chemicals, Healthier Families.* (2018). Retrieved From: http://
saferchemicals.org.

Shutes, Jade. (Accessed 2018, March 6). "The Quality of Essential Oils".
*National Association for Holistic Aromatherapy.* Retrieved from: http://
naha.org/assets/uploads/The_Quality_of_Essential_Oils_Journal.pdf.

The Allergista. (2017, April 3). "Other Names for Propylene Glycol". *The
Allergista.* Retrieved from: http://www.theallergista.com/blog/2017/3/30/
names-for-propylene-glycol.

Villett, Michelle. (2014, October 16). "5 Reasons to Avoid Petroleum and
Mineral Oil in Your Skincare". *Beauty Editor.* Retrieved from: https://
beautyeditor.ca/2014/10/16/petroleum-mineral-oil-skin-products.

*Federal Drug Administration.* (2014, August 22). "Aromatherapy". Retrieved
from: https://www.fda.gov/cosmetics/productsingredients/products/
ucm127054.htm.

# Suggested Resources

Because of my medical background, I am a researcher by nature. When I began using Young Living Essential Oils, I listened to peoples' advice and opinions, but I did my own research as well. Below is a list of books that I have used in my journey to becoming confident with essential oils. This list isn't all-inclusive, but it will provide a good starting point for a beginner.

1. *Gentle Babies: Essential Oils and Natural Remedies for Pregnancy, Childbirth, Infants, and Young Children* by Debra Raybern, www.growinghealthyhomes.com
2. *Healing Oils of the Bible* by David Stewart, www.raindroptraining.com
3. *The Essential Oils Desk Reference*, www.discoverlsp.com
4. *The Essential Oils Pocket Reference*, www.discoverlsp.com
5. *The Chemistry of Essential Oils Made Simple* by David Stewart, www.raindroptraining.com
6. *Essentials: 50 Answers to Common Questions About Essential Oils* by Lindsey Elmore, www.growinghealthyhomes.com

# Notes

# Notes

_____

_____

_____

_____

_____

_____

_____

_____

_____

_____

_____

_____

_____

_____

_____

_____

_____

_____

_____

To obtain additional copies and for more information on other books by Growing Healthy Homes, please visit our website at www.GrowingHealthyHomes.com

## The ABC's of Building a Young Living Organization

## Conquering Toxic Emotions

## Essentials: 50 Answers To Common Questions About Essential Oils

## Gentle Babies

## Road to Royal: Roadmap to Success

# Getting to the
## Water's Edge
## on Whidbey & Camano Islands

THIRD EDITION

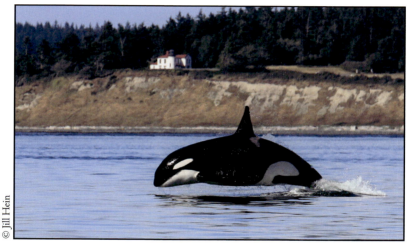

© Jill Hein

## BY SOUND WATER STEWARDS

Trained volunteers working in and around Island County
for a healthy sustainable marine environment through
education, science, and stewardship.

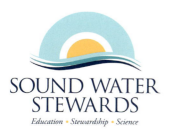

SOUND WATER
STEWARDS
*Education • Stewardship • Science*

*Published by*
**Sound Water Stewards of Island County**
**501(c)(3) non-profit**

**PO Box 1620**
**Freeland, WA 98249**
**soundwaterstewards.org**

Copyright © 2020. Sound Water Stewards of Island County
Third Edition.

Copyright © 1994, 2006. First Edition, Revised (Second) Edition
Washington State University Extension - Island County

All rights reserved. No portion of this book may be used or reproduced in any manner except as
may be expressly permitted by applicable copyright statutes or in writing by the publisher, except
in the case of brief quotations embodied in critical articles or reviews.

ISBN: 978-1-7343529-0-0
Library of Congress Control Number: 2019919404

Recommended citation:
Sound Water Stewards of Island County. 2020. *Getting to the Water's Edge on Whidbey &
Camano Islands*, Third Edition, 208 pages.

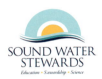

For more information or to learn of updates, contact:

Sound Water Stewards of Island County
PO Box 1620
Freeland, WA 98249
360-678-4401
soundwaterstewards.org

Published February 1, 2020; Second Printing January 3, 2022.
Printed carbon-neutral in Canada on 10% post-consumer recycled stock by Hemlock Printers.
Hemlock is a Forest Stewardship Council® certified printer.
FSC® sets the global gold standard for sustainable forest management.

MIX
Paper from
responsible sources
FSC
www.fsc.org   FSC® C014956

x̌ʷəlč

## The first stewards of the Salish Sea

With the retreat of the Vashon Glacier approximately 12,000 years ago, people came to settle on the shores of the Salish Sea. We can imagine their appreciation for this place with life-filled water everywhere–ocean, inland sea, lakes, rivers, and streams. This water, fresh and salty, intertwined every aspect of their lives. Waterways provided routes to travel. The waters supported an abundance of fish, marine mammals, shellfish, and plants for food. Recognition and gratitude for the water is recorded in Native storytelling, ceremonies, and art. Measures to conserve this rich resource for generations to come were inherent in every aspect of their culture, and promised to sustain their way of life.

Today, with an undercurrent of ecological concern, Coast Salish First People continue to seek solutions and positive actions to secure a healthy Salish Sea. They believe their stewardship now benefits all the residents of this treasured region they have long called home.

x̌ʷəlč *(pronounced roughly "hull-ch") is the native Coast Salish word for saltwater, or the Salish Sea, in the Lushootseed language.*

## Would you join us in stewardship?

The waters, shores, and trails of Whidbey and Camano Islands are in our care for a few short years and then will pass to the next generation and the one after that.

We are stewards with many concerns. We must respect private property, provide public recreational opportunities, protect fragile resources, and enable legitimate commercial, industrial, and agricultural activities. We believe we can, and must, balance them all.

To achieve this balance, we must base more of our daily, personal, and voluntary decisions on our understanding and love of these waters. We must think and act more as stewards–for our own generation and for those who follow.

Please join us.

# Acknowledgements

Many people helped bring this book to life. The vision of Don Meehan, Director of Washington State University Extension—Island County 1982-2008, inspired both the first edition in 1994 and the major revision that followed in 2006. We gratefully acknowledge those who conceived the original Getting to the Water's Edge: Robert Barnes, Larry Landstrom, Susie Nelson, Don Meehan, Cheryl Bradkin, Joyce Terrell, and Doug Dailer.

Special thanks go to Sarah Schmidt, Dan Pedersen, and Stacey Neumiller, the authors of the wonderfully crafted 2006 volume.

Beaches are not static. Wind, time, and especially human actions create changes in our landscape. This third edition updates the content to reflect conditions in 2019-2020 and adds new sites, new essays, and a trail guide. It was produced entirely by Sound Water Steward volunteers, who gave their time and expertise and were assisted by many friends of SWS.

Linda Ade Ridder was project lead. Jordan Macke coordinated ground truthing and initial production work. Sarah Schmidt, lead author of the 2006 edition, served as coordinator for the latter stages of production. Marian Blue created the production copy, edited text, and helped guide the publication process. Cheryl Bradkin was chief editor and the only volunteer who worked on all three editions of GTWE. Lee Badovinus, Kristin Galbreaith, Jeanie McElwain, and Kelly Webb revisited sites, wrote and edited text, and proofread. Bruce McKeown and Freda McKeown copy edited. Kerry Holland and Mariana Noble provided copy editing and created the index.

Every site in this book was visited, photographed, and documented by ground truthers Ron Beier, Barbara Bennett, Bill Bradkin, Barbara Brock, Brenda Dewey, Tom Eisenberg, Kristin Galbreaith, Penny Harger, Shirley Hutchison, Jordan Macke, Jeanie McElwain, PaulBen McElwain, Kathryn McNally, Rachel Nostrom, Linda Ade Ridder, Joan Schrammeck, Charles Seablom, Arlene Stebbins, Michael Stilwell, Stacey Thompson, and Vance Willsey.

Essays are designed to inform and inspire readers to better understand and protect the Island County environment within the context of the larger ecosystem. Dan Pedersen authored many essays carried over from the 2006 edition. Frances Wood contributed bird essays. Mary Allison, Barbara Brock, Paul Hesla, Joan Schrammeck, Val Schroeder, and Stacey Thompson revised Camano essays and gave input on Camano sites and topics. Kristin Galbreaith, Jeanie McElwain, Marian Blue, and Kelly Webb wrote new essays.

Mary Jo Adams and the late Jan Holmes were the original authors of Chapter Four; Mary Jo provided revisions for this edition.

We thank these contributors for updating and expanding Chapter Five: Graham and Shirley Hutchison and Pam Pritzl for birding Camano and Stanwood; Sarah Schmidt for birding Whidbey; Barbara Brock, Dale Christenson, Joan Gerteis, and Phyllis Kind for kayaking routes and advice; Bob Gentz, and Tom Eisenberg of FOCIP for fishing information; Leigh Bloom and Linda Ade Ridder for revisions to clamming, originally written by the late Eugene Thrasher; and Kelly Webb for dog parks. SWS staff Allie Hudec, Joan Schrammeck, and Kelly Zupich wrote about Favorite Beaches with Children. Jeanie McElwain authored information about disability access throughout the book. She and Sarah Schmidt developed the guide to trails in Chapter Six.

Photographers are noted with each photo; we are grateful for the beauty added by their work.

Many friends of Sound Water Stewards also contributed in various ways. Richard Gammon, retired University of Washington faculty, wrote about the global climate crisis. Michele Balagot, Lushootseed Department Manager of Tulalip Tribes, and Jason Ticknor, Archives Manager of Samish Indian Nation, provided insight into native peoples and languages. Susan Berta, Howard Garrett, and Cindy Hansen of Orca Network contributed to the marine mammal sections; Deb Bell and Jeff Wheeler, Washington State Parks, provided input on Cama Beach and Camano Island State Parks.

Patiently answering our questions were Anna Toledo, Island County Marine Resources Committee Project Coordinator; Jim Exe, Island County Health Department; Helen Price Johnson, Island County Commissioner; Karen Bishop, Whidbey Island Conservation District; Ron Newberry, Jessica Larson, and other Whidbey Camano Land Trust staff; Stan Reeves, Executive Director, Port of South Whidbey; Camille Speck, WDFW Lead Biologist for Puget Sound Intertidal Clams and Oyster Fisheries; and Mary Margaret Haugen, Utsalady Ladies Aid.

All funds for printing the book had to be raised in advance. Former SWS Directors Janet St. Clair and Nan Maysen recruited initial sponsors. A team of volunteers picked up where they left off, raising funds and working to market and distribute this book. That committee, led by Jeanie McElwain, includes Kristin Galbreaith, Rachel Nostrom, Joan Schrammeck, Deborah Stilwell, Michael Stilwell, Stacey Thompson, Kelly Webb, John Welsch, and Vance Willsey.

We thank all these wonderful and dedicated women and men who devoted countless hours to share their love and knowledge of the Island County marine environment with you. To any who were overlooked, we apologize sincerely. Come with us now—learn about and explore the wonders of Whidbey and Camano Islands.

# Contents

## CHAPTER ONE

### Before You Go.................................................................... 1

## CHAPTER TWO

### Stewardship in a Warming World........................................ 11

## CHAPTER THREE

### Shoreline Access................................................................ 18

# Whidbey Island Sites

## NORTH WHIDBEY SITES

## CENTRAL WHIDBEY SITES

## SOUTH WHIDBEY SITES

# Camano Island Sites

## CHAPTER FOUR
### Guide to Intertidal Life ............................................................ 125
*Get to know the invertebrates and seaweeds you're most likely to see.*

## CHAPTER FIVE
### Exploring the Edge ................................................................ 135

## CHAPTER SIX
### Guide to Trails ..................................................................... 169
*Trails in Island County.* &#9855; *indicates accessible trails.*

### CAMANO ISLAND TRAILS

# NORTH WHIDBEY ISLAND TRAILS

# CENTRAL WHIDBEY ISLAND TRAILS

# SOUTH WHIDBEY ISLAND TRAILS

# SITE TABLE

# SITE MAP

# INDEX

# SPONSORS

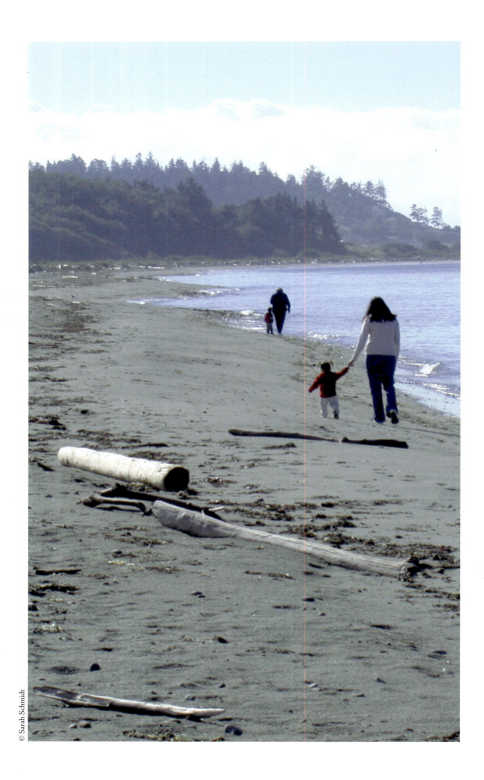

© Sarah Schmidt

# CHAPTER ONE

# *Before You Go*

## Safety is your responsibility

This isn't a safety handbook.

As you read and use this book, please understand that safety is solely your responsibility. We want to help you enjoy the outdoors but cannot assure that these sites, trails, beaches, waterways, or activities are safe for all individuals at all times and in all conditions. You're responsible for knowing your limitations. Prepare wisely, assess conditions, have the right equipment, understand emergency procedures, and avoid unnecessary risks. **Users of this book assume responsibility and all risks** for any loss, injury or death that might result from the activities described or from using the maps and information presented.

All recreation involves hazards. These include, for example, overexertion, equipment failure, changing weather, tides, currents, marine traffic, shellfish poisoning, chemicals in treated lumber, toxic waste or biological matter, obstacles, shifting logs, earth-slide, poor visibility, unsafe footing, and falling debris.

A sincere effort has been made to minimize errors in the data, maps and other information in this book. However, conditions change over time and some errors might have been missed. Therefore, Sound Water Stewards and those working with that organization are absolved from all risks incurred from relying upon the information in this book.

## Tidelands – the issue of private ownership

Washington's constitution, adopted in 1889, followed the precedent of earlier states and claimed ownership of all beds and shores of navigable waters up to and including the line of ordinary high water (mean high tide). Consequently, all tidelands in the state were public tidelands.

The state made no provision for the owners of upland property to gain access to saltwater for shipping, to propagate fish or shellfish, or to engage in other marine-related industry. To provide access for these activities and to generate revenue, the Washington Legislature authorized the sale of public tidelands to private individuals. Since then, the state sold about 60 percent of public tidelands to private owners before discontinuing this practice in 1967. Because of those sales in Island County, about half of all tidelands are privately owned.

### Rights on private tidelands

We strongly urge the public to use **public access** to reach **public tidelands;** respect private property at all times. Sites in this book were selected on public accessibility. It's illegal to trespass on **privately owned** uplands.

Does this mean the public can or can't cross privately owned tidelands for the purpose of getting to publicly owned tidelands?

The Public Trust Doctrine (a legal principle, which is part of U.S. common law but not statutory law) states that all waters of our state are owned by and available to all citizens equally. This principle affords certain access rights but is complicated and subject to testing and interpretation in courts. Its interpretation under Washington law simply isn't clear.

What is clear is that private tidelands, uplands, and all other private property must be respected. Unlike upland properties, tidelands often have no fencing to mark boundaries. In this book, we indicate the length of public tidelands when available, but you won't find any signs marking the property lines unless put there by private-tideland owners.

Good faith efforts were made to work with local jurisdictions to verify the extent of public tideland for the 2020 third edition of this publication. No public tidelands have been sold since the previous edition, so the measurements are deemed as accurate as possible. However, please be aware that over time, as land shifts from one property owner to the next, it's not uncommon for the official boundary line between public and private land to become blurred. Without an official and recent survey there is almost never a way to tell where the actual boundary line is, and thus it's best to always err on the side of caution and turn around before treading on private land.

Always obtain permission from private property owners before you remain on or take anything from their property. For instance, it's illegal to take shellfish from private tidelands without the owner's permission.

### To get there legally for sure...

This book identifies dozens of locations where the public may gain legal access to public tidelands. **Tidelands** are the parts of a beach alternately covered and uncovered by the rising and falling tides. **Uplands** are the parts above the high tide mark, which almost always remain dry but may be partially covered during extremely high tides or storms.

The distinctions are important. Even though the tidelands at a certain location may be publicly owned, the upland parts may be privately owned.

In Island County, almost all the upland parts of beaches are privately owned. The public owns and can use about half of the tidelands. The problem is that many stretches of public tidelands can't be reached from land without trespassing on private uplands.

All the public tidelands listed in this publication can be reached by a public road ending at or next to publicly owned upland access. Many of the upland accesses are quite narrow. Tideland users should know that if they leave a public beach access where the tidelands are public and walk along the beach in either direction, sooner or later they will reach private tidelands. **These are not likely to be marked with a sign.** For example, a 50-foot-wide public road may provide access to only 50 feet of public upland and tideland; alternatively, it may provide access to more than a mile of public tidelands In the latter case, except for the upland at the road end, the whole stretch of upland is probably private.

On any beach, the amount of tideland exposed and available for walking or other use will, of course, change as the tides rise and fall during the day. If you walk near the water's edge at any time other than a few hours before or after a high tide, you are probably on the tidelands. However, if you are on a beach at any time near high tide you may well be on the upland. Unless you know differently, you should assume you are on private property, and it's illegal to remain on or take anything from private property without the property owner's permission.

### *Uplands—look for the wrack line*

Generally, most public tidelands begin at ordinary high tide, also called the **mean high tide.** This is defined as the average of all high tides for the last 19 years and can range from 7.1 feet at Neah Bay to 13.5 feet at Olympia. The graphic that follows on the next page depicts the various tides. Notice that mean high tide is lower than extreme high tide.

High tides often leave a wrack line (a line of natural detris, such as feathers, shell fragments, sea vegetation) on the beach at the water's highest point. The wrack line conveniently provides a guide between public tideline and private uplands. If you've ventured onto the crest of the beach and are walking on the large drift logs that have been there for years, you are almost certainly above the mean high tide level and, in most cases, will be trespassing on private uplands. On some beaches there may be multiple wrack lines. This is especially likely to occur during low tide events in the summer. Your best bet is to stay as comfortably close to the lowest wrack line as you can without sinking in tidal mudflats.

To complicate matters, upland ownership of many waterfront properties in Island County was granted prior to statehood and extends to the **meander line.** The meander line is the original surveyed shoreline rather than a constant elevation line, so naturally occurring erosion and accretion make the upland boundary lines subject to constant change. In some places the meander line is now on dry land, but in many cases it may be some distance offshore from the line of mean high tide. There is no easy way to locate such a line by examining the beach for the wrack line.

Perhaps the best rule is that if you walk near the water's edge at any time other than within a few hours of the high tide of the day, you're probably not trespassing on uplands. Please remember that at high tide, it may be impossible to walk on public tidelands. It's your responsibility to know where you are and when you're there.

**TIDE LEVEL DIAGRAM**
(From WDFW Shellfish Regs. website)

**UPLAND**
(Usually Private Ownership)

**TIDELAND**
(Public or Private Ownership)

**BEDLAND**
(Public Ownership)

| | |
|---|---|
| Extreme High Tide | +11.0 ft. |
| Mean High Tide | +6.6 ft. |
| Mean Low Tide | +2.5 ft. |
| Mean Lower Low Tide | 0.0 ft. |
| Extreme Low Tide | -4.0 ft. |

## Park with courtesy

When parking at a public beach access, please be considerate. Obey the posted signs explaining the parking rules. They are supported by state, county, and city ordinances. If you're caught in violation of these ordinances you'll be subject to a traffic fine.

For parking at a beach access where no signs designating parking are posted, follow these rules laid out in state law and found in the Washington Driver Guide:

1.  Drivers are responsible for making sure their vehicles aren't a hazard when parked. Be sure to park in a place that's far enough from any travel lane to avoid interfering with traffic and that's also visible to vehicles approaching from either direction.

2.  Do not park
    *   in front of or within five feet of a public or private driveway, alley, or private road.
    *   within 15 feet of a fire hydrant.

- within 20 feet of a pedestrian safety zone.
- within 30 feet of a traffic signal, stop sign, yield sign, or any similar traffic control device.

These are just some of the more likely applicable motor vehicle regulations. Others may be found in the online guide at **dol.wa.gov.** A general guideline is to be courteous and to respect the needs of others, including the adjoining property owners.

## If physical mobility is a challenge…

Soft sand, logs, rocks, steep slopes, and other barriers may make getting to the water's edge difficult or impossible for persons with many kinds of mobility challenges.

We highlight some beach accesses that have various degrees of accessibility. Few will get you exactly to the water's edge, but many will get you near. You'll often find that you can walk or wheel to at least the upland edge of the beach, to viewpoints, or even over the water on some piers. At many sites, you can also enjoy the sights, smells, and sounds of the beach from the safety and comfort of your car.

Find these beaches in Chapter Five (see pgs. 159-164). These include ADA-styled restrooms, handicapped parking, picnic areas, shelters, piers, trails, and more. The site descriptions in Chapter Three will tell you more about what is available at each beach.

Above all, remember that your safety is your responsibility. Since types of challenges to mobility are so varied, an "accessible site" may not meet the needs of everyone. If you choose to use soft paths, piers, ramps, floats, or other kinds of unstable or steep surfaces, be very alert to their possible dangers to you. Some persons with challenges advise taking a partner who can help out with barriers such as heavy bathroom doors and who can also assess the challenges on that beach on that day since the conditions on beaches can change drastically and quickly.

## Beach safety

Every year people underestimate beach hazards and require rescue or recovery because they were trapped by the tide, injured, or killed. Beach safety is your responsibility. Please keep these following points in mind.

**Tides and bluffs:** Be especially cautious when beach walking in high bluff areas. Often these areas offer no accessible upland beach for retreat from rising tides. Tides in the Northwest are asymmetrical, meaning the day's two high tides (and two lows) can be of greatly different heights, unlike the East Coast where they are nearly identical. You can be trapped by the incoming tide. To avoid this on a high bluff beach, you must be aware of the daily tides.

**Climbing:** Please do not climb on fragile bluffs. This can go wrong in all kinds of ways including falls and landslides. Keep children and pets clear of these areas as well.

**Shoes:** Wear shoes or boots that provide a good grip. Use caution on slippery rocks. The barnacles and other hard-shelled animals found on rocks can be razor sharp.

**Hazardous litter:** Take precautions when picking up litter. Wearing gloves is a good idea. Do not touch questionable items such as hypodermic needles, dangerous waste, or containers of possibly hazardous materials. Note their location and notify the Island County Sheriff or the Island County Health Department. (See contact numbers on pg. 9.)

**Shellfish:** Before gathering shellfish, recreational harvesters should seek current information about Paralytic Shellfish Poisoning (PSP) from the Island County Health Department (see pg. 9) or the State PSP Hotline (800-562-5632) or search online for "island county WA shellfish" and "WA department of health recreational shellfish." Shellfish harvesters should always remember to fill their digging holes.

**Swimming:** The water temperature in the Salish Sea ranges from 45°F in the winter to 55°F in the summer. Tidal changes create strong rip tides that challenge the strongest swimmers. For swimming beach advisories, search online for "WA department of health swimming beaches Whidbey Island."

Chapter Three includes many site descriptions that detail swimming opportunities.

## Beach fires – what you must know

Current rules on beach fires (Recreational Burning) are covered under Outdoor Burning Permit Information available on the Island County or Northwest Clean Air Agency websites. At times all outdoor burning is restricted or banned, and there are some areas that have permanent no burning designations.

In Island County, recreational fires don't need a permit if all conditions below are met. Check for additional restrictions in your area.

- The fire must consist of only charcoal or firewood and must be used only for cooking or pleasure.
- Winds must be less than 7 mph.
- The fire must be 3 feet in diameter or smaller and be in an enclosure no larger than 3 feet across. The enclosure must be a minimum of 16 inches high and made of cement block, stones, or 10-gauge steel.

- Materials being burned must be kept lower than the sidewalls of the enclosure.
- A charged garden hose or two five-gallon buckets of water, as well as a shovel or rake, must be on site.
- The fire must be 25 feet from any structure or standing timber.
- Tree branches must be cleared to a height of 15 feet above the enclosure.
- One person age 16 or older, who is capable of putting the fire out, must be in attendance at all times and must have a way to call 911.
- The fire must be contained within a firebreak (bare ground).
- The landowner's permission must be obtained if not on your property, and the fire must not create a nuisance.
- Fires must be fully extinguished, wet, and cold to the touch when departing the beach area.

For more information, call the Island County Public Health Department during business hours: on Whidbey Island, 360-679-7350; on Camano Island, 360-678-8261.

## How to explore the beach without harming it

Low tides provide ample opportunities to explore the beach and discover all the fascinating creatures normally hidden from view. It's important to remember that at low tides these animals and plants are especially vulnerable. They are exposed not only to sun and predators but also to us. We can easily damage them or their habitat.

We teach our children important lifetime values when we instill an ethic of respect and stewardship toward all life. Beach animals and plants thrive best if we leave them alone. With care, we can minimize the risk to living creatures as we foster the sense of wonder that comes from touching a sea star's rough "skin," feeling a hermit crab crawl on our hands, or looking eye-to-tentacle with an enormous moon snail.

*We recommend the following beach etiquette be observed by adults and children:*

- **Walk with care** to avoid injuring plants and animals—life is under your feet. Beach plants prevent erosion. Seaweeds are living blankets that provide habitat and hiding places for many animals, keeping them safe from air, sun, and predators. Eelgrass beds are plant and animal nurseries. Step on bare spots if you can.
- **Kneel quietly by tidepools** and try to not walk in them.
- **Overturn rocks and blades of eelgrass with care** and with a clean hand and then return them softly to their original position to avoid crushing the animals or leaving them exposed to the elements or pred-

ators. Lift only rocks that can be moved with one hand. Rock undersides are marine condominiums. If the animals that live there are left uncovered, you destroy their home and possibly them, too.

- **Touch animals gently** and avoid handling all soft-bodied animals altogether. Touch animals only with a clean finger that is moistened in sea water. Sea stars are usually durable on their upper surface, but if you touch their tube feet, they may attach to your skin and then be torn when you remove them.

- **Enjoy anemones** without prodding them. Anemones often squirt water if poked, but this can kill them because they need that water to stay wet until the next tide covers them.

- **Leave alone attached animals** such as anemones, barnacles, and mussels. Pulling and prying them from rocks or pilings will kill them.

- **Marine mammals such as baby seals must be left alone.** They're protected by the Marine Mammal Protection Act. Always keep a safe distance (minimum of 100 yards) away because most likely the mother is off hunting for food and will return, sometimes hours or days later.

- **Fill any holes you dig.** Leave clams and other organisms at the same depth and in the same orientation as you found them. Piles of sand left on the beach can smother organisms beneath.

- **Leave the beach clean.** Bring a litterbag and carry out your own garbage as well as any trash you find, especially plastics, which are hazards to a variety of marine life and birds.

- **Prevent pets** from harassing wildlife; always carry out your pet's wastes.

- **Obtain permits** before harvesting any animals or plants. Obey limits set by fish and game laws.

## How we sized up the sites

People use public beach accesses in many different ways, so we tried to include what you might need to know. For instance, a restroom and drinking water are important to most, but if you're gathering a group, you may also need ample parking and picnic tables, barbecue grills, and a playground. If trailering a big boat, you'll need a worthy ramp, but if kayaking, you may require only a gravelly beach on which to hand-carry boats to the water. We point out beach-walking opportunities for sites with 600 or more feet of public tidelands. We also indicate which sites have wheelchair-accessible facilities: ♿. We also indicate sites often used for swimming, shore casting, and bird watching. Whether your goal is to enjoy the view from a parked car or explore miles of public shoreline, you'll find what you're seeking on these pages.

# Phone numbers to keep handy

Phone numbers change often, so if these don't work, check the websites for County, State, and Federal agencies. If you like, record the new number in your book. Agencies referenced below are Washington Departments of Fish and Wildlife (WDFW), Health (WDOH), Natural Resources (WDNR), and National Oceanographic and Atmospheric Administration (NOAA).

| | |
|---|---|
| 9-1-1 | Emergencies – fire, ambulance, police |
| 360-678-4422 | Sheriff, Island County from north, central Whidbey |
| 360-321-5113 | Sheriff, Island County from south Whidbey, x 7310 |
| 360-629-4523 | Sheriff, Island County from Camano Island, x 7310 |
| 855-542-3935 | Derelict fishing gear, poaching or dangerous wildlife, WDFW |
| 800-853-1964 | Enforcement hotline, National Marine Fisheries Service |
| 360-236-4501 | Fish consumption advisories, WDOH |
| 866-246-9453 | Fishing and hunting license sales, WDFW |
| 360-902-2500 | Fishing rule change hotline |
| 360-678-2349 | Island County Marine Resources Committee |
| 360-679-7335 | Island County Parks and Trails |
| 360-679-7350 | Island County Public Health from Whidbey |
| 360-678-8261 | Island County Public Health from Camano |
| 800-853-1964 | Marine mammal harassment, NOAA |
| 360-678-3765 | Marine mammal dead or stranded – Island County |
| 877-767-9425 | Marine mammal entanglements hotline |
| 866-672-2638 | Marine mammal stranded, Orca Network |
| 360-428-1617 | NW Clean Air Agency |
| 800-258-5990 | Oil or chemical spills, WA Emergency Management |
| 800-222-4737 | Oiled birds, WDFW |
| 866-672-2638 | Orca whale sightings, Orca Network |
| 800-562-5632 | Shellfish Safety/Paralytic Shellfish Poisoning Hotline, WDOH |
| 866-880-5431 | Shellfish rule change hotline, licenses, WDFW |
| 360-678-4401 | Sound Water Stewards of Island County |
| 888-226-7688 | Washington State Parks Camping Reservations |
| 360-902-8844 | Washington State Parks Information (M-F 8 AM to 5 PM) |
| 425-775-1311 | WDFW North Puget Sound office |
| 360-791-9555 | Whale stranding hotline, Cascadia Research Collective |
| 800-562-6010 | Wildfires and woodcutting, WDNR |

# MARINE STEWARDSHIP AREAS

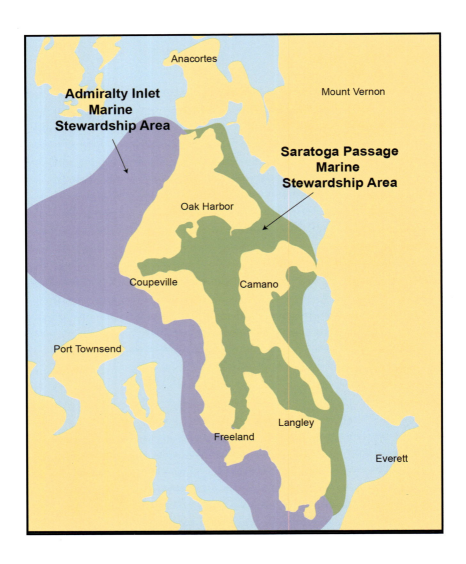

# CHAPTER TWO

## *Stewardship in a warming world*

### The global climate emergency

Rapid global climate change is here. Global warming–increasing average global surface temperature due to human emissions of greenhouse gases–is changing every part of the planet, including our Pacific Northwest.

Global warming is caused by a well-understood natural process—the greenhouse effect, which refers to the heat-trapping capacity of several trace gases in Earth's atmosphere, most importantly carbon dioxide ($CO_2$), methane ($CH_4$), and water vapor ($H_2O$); these primarily come from fossil fuel burning (coal, oil, and natural gas). Visible sunlight warms the earth, and the warmed earth and atmosphere send heat to space. But greenhouse gases capture some of the outgoing heat radiated from Earth's surface and atmosphere, redirecting this heat energy back down toward the surface, warming our planet.

The heat-trapping ability of several of these trace gases was demonstrated in the laboratory more than 150 years ago. In the 1890s, a Swedish scientist predicted that Earth would warm about 9°F if the atmospheric $CO_2$ concentration were doubled. At the presently observed rate of $CO_2$ increase, we will reach this predicted doubling in this century. The observed global surface temperature record can now be attributed with overwhelming confidence (more than 3 million to one) to our greenhouse gas emissions.

No living person has ever breathed this anticipated atmospheric $CO_2$ level, nor has any human who ever lived, back to the first *Homo sapiens* arising in Africa 200,000 years ago. Only our primitive ancestors of 3.5 million years ago breathed this level of $CO_2$, when the global temperature was 4-6° F warmer than now, and the sea level was 40-60 feet higher. If emissions continue to escalate, the results are likely to be far worse.

Over 90% of the excess warming is being absorbed by the global surface ocean. Ocean waters, now more acidic from absorbing a third of our $CO_2$ emissions, are also "breathless" because warmer waters hold less oxygen. Warmer ocean waters are killing marine species or are forcing them to retreat toward the poles. Half of the world's tropical coral reefs have already died due to coral bleaching associated with higher ocean temperatures and acidity. We have entered the sixth mass extinction with entire species disappearing from the far reaches of our planet, both above and below its waters.

Nothing in our history has prepared us for such rapid and catastrophic changes in Earth's climate.

Warming will be greater at higher latitudes than near the equator, on land than over the ocean, in winter than in summer, and at night than during the day...exactly as now observed. Melting ice with the resulting sea level rise and changes in precipitation patterns are predicted to impact life on Earth more adversely than just warming temperatures. Weather (atmospheric conditions over a short period of time) will be even more extreme, with more powerful hurricanes, greater rainfall and flooding, and drier and longer droughts. At higher latitudes, glaciers will continue to disappear and snowpack will decline. Summer arctic sea ice may disappear entirely. Increasingly rapid loss of polar ice sheets in Greenland and West Antarctica is already causing acceleration of global sea level rise.

Global climate change impacts—such as hotter summers with prolonged periods of drought, reduced snowpack, and more winter flooding—are also affecting the Pacific Northwest, though less extremely than at lower latitudes. Forest fires will increase on both sides of the Cascades. Trees are dying from insect infestation, disease, and drought. Ocean acidification, which reduces the uptake of calcium in marine species, is damaging our coasts' shellfish. Our salmon runs, beloved orcas, and gray whales are threatened with starvation and even extinction.

Rising sea level and storm surges in this century will impact thousands of our coastal properties at the high tide line. And, because the impacts will be much worse in other parts of this country and throughout the world, we in the Pacific Northwest can expect a major influx of climate migrants and refugees.

What can we do? Each of us can study climate science; talk about the climate emergency with our families, neighbors, and colleagues; and work to reduce our own additions to the $CO_2$ in our atmosphere. We can begin to prepare now for those fleeing regions that are becoming uninhabitable. We can mobilize support for climate change mitigation and adaptation policies at all levels: at home, in our towns, counties, state, nation, and world. Most of all, we can aim for a carbon-neutral world with no net increase in greenhouse gas emissions by 2050 or earlier. Our collective actions are critical, but whether you are a resident or a visitor to our islands, your individual actions are becoming increasingly important.

## Stewardship is more important than ever

All of the beaches and natural areas described in this book were home to indigenous peoples for tens of thousands of years. They traveled the waterways, camped, and lived on beaches and shores. They harvested berries, cedar bark and roots, and other food, including clams, crabs, and salmon provided by the waters and beaches. They lived harmoniously with nature and were good stewards of the resources. Their actions did not adversely impact the climate.

For better or worse, we are now the stewards of the Island County natural world for generations to come. The condition in which we leave the natural world is our legacy. Stewardship is about accepting personal responsibility to learn about, respect, and preserve that which is in our trust. Our lives depend on clean water and a healthy environment.

## What you can do

As you explore and enjoy the waters and woods of Whidbey and Camano Islands, please remember that you are not the first nor the last to visit. Be a good steward of our beaches, trails, and marine life. Learn all you can. Observe carefully. Be sure that your actions help, rather than harm, the animals, plants, and their environment. Understand that you are preserving them for future generations. Help others understand, as well.

## Become a Sound Water Steward

One of the best ways to learn about our shores and marine life is to become a Sound Water Stewards trained volunteer. This program was founded by the Washington State University Cooperative Extension Program Director for Island County in 1989 as Beach Watchers. In 2016, the Beach Watchers program left the WSU umbrella to become an independent non-profit corporation with the same mission, goals, and volunteers.

This fascinating and deeply satisfying educational program will enrich your life. Sound Water Stewards receive over 100 hours of classroom and field training in a wide range of topics including forestry, coastal geology, marine biology, watersheds, beach monitoring, marine estuaries, and climate impact.

In return for this education, trained Sound Water Stewards make a commitment to give back to the community. They share their knowledge by performing at least 100 hours of service in community outreach programs, fulfilling the mission of Sound Water Stewards of Island County:

*to provide trained volunteers working in and around Island County for a healthy, sustainable Puget Sound environment through education, community outreach, stewardship, and citizen science.*

For more information or to apply to become a Sound Water Steward please visit **info@soundwaterstewards.org**.

## Become a Shore Steward

Shore Stewards is another educational program developed by WSU Extension. The free, voluntary program is offered to homeowners, landowners, businesses, farms, cities, marinas, parks, and others located along any waterfront, lake, or stream—i.e., along a shoreline. For information or to receive a guide, visit the Island County Shore Stewards website: **extension.wsu.edu/island/nrs/shore-stewards** or call 360-639-4608.

Shore Stewards voluntarily follow nature-friendly practices in caring for their beaches, bluffs, and property.

**Ten simple but important guidelines** help create and preserve a healthy shoreline environment for fish, wildlife, and birds as well as people:

- Take care of waste from people, pets, and products, including regularly inspecting and maintaining septic systems.
- Work with nature by maintaining a buffer on the water's edge to minimize run-off and protect your trees.
- Make wise choices when landscaping by using native plants, by controlling weeds and pests safely, and by composting whenever possible.
- Manage water runoff and use low impact development to prevent pollution.
- Reduce erosion and landslide risk through plantings and other natural solutions, as well as removing bulkheads.
- For those living along lakes and streams, take care to minimize the run-off of animal waste, fertilizers, and chemicals.
- When boating, preserve clean water by preventing pollution and fuel spills, protecting eelgrass habitat, preventing the spread of invasive species, watching whales and other marine life from a safe distance, and learning how to crab responsibly.
- Conserve water in your home and garden.
- Respect intertidal life while you have fun on the beach and as you harvest fish and shellfish.
- Learn what you need to know before you build or clear land near the shore.

Whether or not you choose to be a Shore Steward, we hope you will follow these good stewardship practices. In addition to protecting the environment and property, many find it can result in higher property values.

# Marine Resources Committee

Since 1999, efforts to understand and protect the diversity of life in our shoreline waters have been led by citizen-based Marine Resources Committees (MRCs) in all seven coastal counties of northern Puget Sound. These committees report to their local county commissioners and to the Northwest Straits Commission, which was established under federal legislation co-sponsored by U.S. Senator Patty Murray and Congressman Jack Metcalf.

Island County MRC brings together scientists, business people, farmers, educators, recreational boaters, sport anglers, lawyers, county employees, port commissioners, and federal government representatives in this shared effort. The Island County MRC has mapped, photographed, and videotaped every foot of Island County's 212 miles of shoreline. They have compiled a comprehensive database of critical eelgrass beds, forage fish spawning beaches, shoreline hardening features, and feeder bluffs. They work in close cooperation with the Island County Salmon Recovery Program to protect and restore nearshore habitats and also with other county committees and departments concerned about water quality, such as the Water Resources Advisory Committee (WRAC) and Salmon Technical Advisory Group (Salmon TAG).

More information may be found at the websites for Island County Marine Resources Committee and for the Northwest Straits Commission.

# Saratoga Passage and Admiralty Inlet Marine Stewardship Areas

Three large marine stewardship areas encompass all Island County waters, including both Whidbey and Camano Islands (see map pg. 10). County leaders created the Saratoga Passage and Admiralty Inlet stewardship areas in 2003 to encourage the public to learn all they can about voluntary stewardship and how to practice it in their day-to-day use of our beaches, waters, and uplands.

In 2013 and 2014, Commissioners in Island and Snohomish counties adopted resolutions in their respective counties to create the Port Susan Marine Stewardship Area. The website of the Island County Marine Resources Committee contains extensive information on all three Stewardship areas. Stewardship area designation calls upon local citizens and visitors to focus increased efforts on understanding and caring for these areas.

### Saratoga Passage Marine Stewardship Area

The Saratoga Passage Marine Stewardship Area designation recognizes its vital importance to salmon, forage fish, and other marine life. The waters between Camano and Whidbey Islands provide a rich and relatively low-energy marine environment of extensive eelgrass beds and small coastal lagoons, providing shelter for juvenile salmon; spawning beaches for forage fish; and ghost shrimp beds, an important feeding area for gray whales. Three major salmon-producing rivers – the Skagit, Stillaguamish, and Snohomish – feed into these waters.

### Admiralty Inlet Marine Stewardship Area

The way in which whales, salmon, trout, and other migratory fish and birds use Whidbey Island's western shoreline is the focus of increasing study by several organizations. This exposed shoreline is one of the highest-energy marine environments in Puget Sound, including heavily-trafficked shipping lanes, a major migration corridor for salmon entering and leaving Puget Sound, and a number of estuaries that provide critical shelter.

### Port Susan Marine Stewardship Area

Port Susan Bay, located between the east side of Camano Island and the Snohomish County mainland, holds some of the finest estuarine habitat in Puget Sound. Port Susan's marshes, tidally influenced channels, and vast mudflats support several species of salmon, smelt, shellfish, and English sole.

## It will take us all

The future health and productivity of our waters will be determined by millions of individual decisions made by hundreds of thousands of residents and visitors. It is neither possible nor desirable to control all those decisions with laws. Education, public understanding, and voluntary behavior change are essential in shaping the legacy our generation will leave for the next.

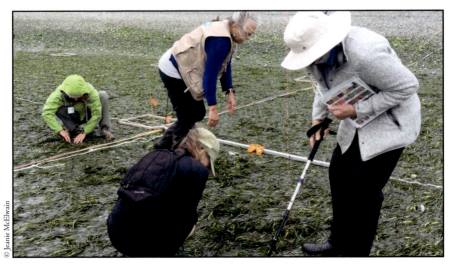

*Intertidal Monitoring at Possession Beach (See Site 57)*

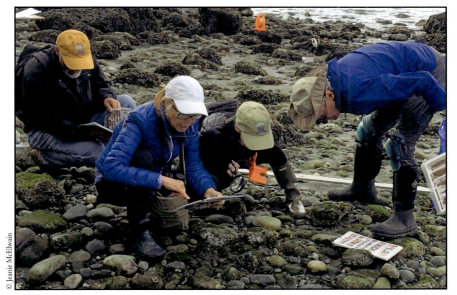

© Jeanie McElwain

*Intertidal Monitoring at Lagoon Point South (see Site 36B)*

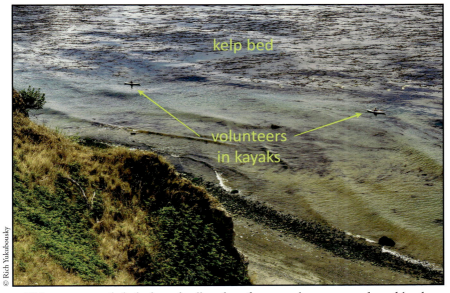

kelp bed

volunteers
in kayaks

© Rich Yakubousky

*Volunteers map kelp beds and collect data for annual surveys conducted by the Island County Marine Resources Committee (pg. 15). Bull kelp forests are important habitats for all types of marine animals critical to the food web (see box pg. 49-50).*

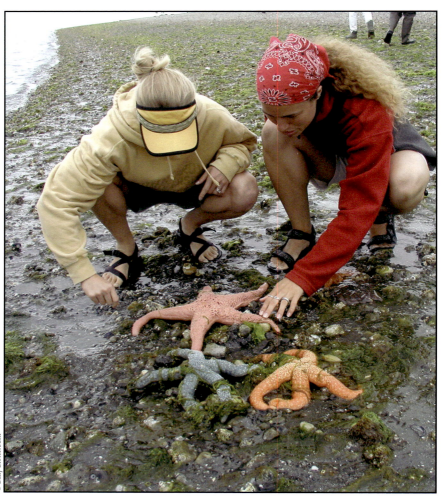

© Sally Slotterback

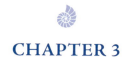

## CHAPTER 3

# *Shoreline Access*

### What we left out

This book doesn't list every access to public tidelands. Some are left out due to inadequate parking, safety concerns, or difficult access. For information on public shoreline access sites not shown here, contact the Island County Planning and Community Development Department. Public tidelands accessible only from the water also are omitted. Check the Washington Department of Natural Resources website for the location of these tidelands.

### Tides can prevent access

At high tide, many sites listed in this book don't allow access to beach walking on adjoining public tideland because high water reaches either private upland or the foot of a bluff. At low tide, exposed mud or sand flats at some sites may make it impossible to launch either trailered or hand-carried boats.

### Finding the sites

To locate the sites listed in this book, use the map on pages 188-189 and the directions listed in the description for each site. We give driving instructions from Highway 20 and Highway 525 for Whidbey and from Terry's Corner for Camano. Visitors will find it helpful to refer to a driving map, online or available from Chambers of Commerce, visitor centers, realtors, and many grocery stores. We abbreviate left, right, north, south, east, and west as L, R, N, S, E, and W.

### Site descriptions

**Coordinates:** We include latitude and longitude coordinates for use with GPS units to help boaters find the public access when approaching from the water. They are intended as a helpful guide. Do not rely on them for safe navigation.

**Parking: 1, 2, 3, 4-6, etc.** indicate parking for this number of vehicles. Sites with boat ramps offer limited parking for boat trailers. Most sites are restricted to day use only. Overnight parking is available in major state parks. Public boat ramps and marinas may charge for launching or parking; check for fees and time limits before planning a trip. To park at a Department of Fish & Wildlife access or state park, you must post a Discover Pass parking permit on your vehicle (except where access is managed by South Whidbey Parks and Recreation). Permits are available online, wherever hunting and fishing licenses are sold, or at state parks.

**Restroom availability** varies by site. Even when flush or non-flush toilets are on a site, they may be closed—at night, seasonally, for maintenance, or for a variety of reasons. Please plan accordingly.

**Symbols for amenities and activities:**

- Restroom with flush toilet.
- Non-flush toilet (either portable or vault toilet).
- Potable water.
- Picnic table(s).
- Covered picnic area.
- Barbecue grill(s) or fire pit.
- Playground.
- Dock or pier. Some are seasonal.
- Boat launch ramp, usable for both trailered and car-top boats. If site has a boat ramp, symbol for hand-carried boat isn't shown.
- No boat ramp is available, but car-top boats such as canoes and kayaks could be hand carried to water's edge. At sites with mudflats, water is reachable only at high tides.
- At least 600 feet of public tideland available for beach walking.
- A site considered a swimming beach.
- A site used for fishing from shore.
- A good site for bird watching.
- Upland hiking trails at site.
- Scenic view from parking area.

Use the Site Table on pages 184-187 to find which sites offer each of these features.

**Adjoining public tideland:** This distance in linear feet indicates how far you can move along the beach before reaching private tideland. We researched this using county property records and descriptions, but the authors, publishers, and sponsors can't guarantee its accuracy. We did not conduct boundary surveys.

# WHIDBEY ISLAND SITES

Forty-five miles long and up to 10 miles wide, Whidbey is the longest island in the contiguous 48 states since a 1985 U.S. Supreme Court decision ruled that New York State's Long Island is actually a peninsula.

Whidbey is reached at its northern end by the Deception Pass Bridge on Highway 20; at its center by the Port Townsend/Coupeville ferry; and at the southern end by the Mukilteo/Clinton ferry on Highway 525. Highway 525 and Highway 20 meet south of Coupeville at Wanamaker Road (called Race Road east of the highway). At this intersection, Highway 525 ends and Highway 20 turns west on Wanamaker Road to the Port Townsend/Coupeville ferry landing at Keystone. Site directions on Whidbey Island are given from Highways 20 and 525, which form the major north-south travel corridor.

## NORTH WHIDBEY

**Site 1**

### DECEPTION PASS STATE PARK
Lat/Long: North Beach 48.4017, -122.6615
West Beach 48.3994, -122.6647

**Directions:** Turn W off Hwy 20 at traffic light 1 mile S of Deception Pass Bridge for the main park entrance, opposite Cornet Bay Rd; there are also entrances at Bowman Bay, Rosario Beach, and Cornet Bay.

**Parking**: 228 at West Beach and many more throughout the park. A Discover Pass is required to park here.

Deception Pass State Park comprises 3,854 acres in Island and Skagit counties and is Washington's most popular state park. It offers a breathtaking bridge, old growth forest, over 300 campsites, 10 kitchen shelters, two freshwater lakes, 10 boat ramps, 14 miles of shoreline, 40 miles of trails and kayaking, bird watching, clamming, crabbing, fresh and saltwater swimming, scuba diving, fishing, sandy beaches, rugged cliffs, and stunning views.

In addition to the Whidbey Island sites described here, the park includes water access north of Deception Pass Bridge at Pass Lake, Bowman Bay, and Rosario Head. Saltwater moorage is available at Cornet Bay and Bowman Bay.

In the 1930s, the Civilian Conservation Corps (CCC) built many of the roads, trails, buildings, and bridges to develop the park. Some of the park trails are near steep banks and cliffs, so carefully attend children.

When exploring the beaches of Deception Pass, keep in mind that six million feet walk the park each year. See how to explore without harming the environment on pg. 7. Enjoy being a steward of the treasures nature created.

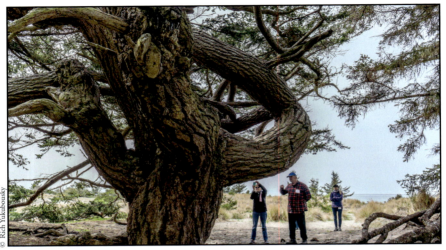

*Ancient tree on Dune Trail, Deception Pass State Park*

## Joseph Whidby

Just over 200 years ago Captain George Vancouver sailed into Puget Sound on the HMS Discovery. He anchored near Mukilteo and sent his ship's master, Joseph Whidby, to explore the inland waters that Europeans later named Port Susan, Saratoga Passage, and Skagit Bay. After exploring these inside waters, Whidby explored waters to the west.

On June 10, 1792, he found a narrow, rocky channel leading into Skagit Bay, which he had explored earlier from the inside. This confirmed he had been circumnavigating an island (which, of course, had been known to indigenous people for millennia). Vancouver 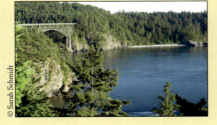 named it Whidby Island (later Whidbey) to honor the officer who identified it. He named the narrow opening Deception Pass. The Swinomish people called the pass *xčiuz*, meaning dangerous.

## CORNET BAY COUNTY DOCK
Lat/Long: 48.3970, -122.6313
288 West Cornet Bay Rd, Oak Harbor

**Directions:** At traffic light 1 mile S of Deception Pass Bridge, turn E onto Cornet Bay Rd. County dock is 1 mile on L at intersection of Cornet Bay Rd and Bay View Ln.

**Parking:** 10 🚻 ♿ ⚓ 🚤

**Adjoining public tideland:** 50 feet, lot width only.

Island County maintains this 120-foot dock for public moorage and hand-launching small boats. Day use only.

For more information search online for "Cornet Bay county docks."

---

### Battle on the beach—intertidal zonation

Intertidal marine creatures on shorelines around the world must cope with a host of physical and biological challenges. As a result, they are grouped into distinct bands or zones. Intertidal zonation is most obvious on steep or rock-faced beaches where the horizontal tide range is small and the bands are narrow. It's less evident on flat beaches where the horizontal tide range can stretch hundreds of feet. Zonation occurs partly because of local tidal conditions and partly because of the evolutionary and ecological makeup of individual plants and animals.

In general, quality of life in the upper tide zones depends on an animal's ability to manage physical conditions such as drying, temperature swings, fresh water dilution, and wave action. In the lower tide zones, the community is determined more by biological factors such as predators and the contest for space, food, and mates.

Four common intertidal invertebrates (spineless creatures) illustrate how zonation works. Very high in the intertidal, a tiny brown barnacle, *Chthamalus*, can take greater exposure to air and changing temperatures than most other invertebrates. It can also thrive much lower in the intertidal but isn't found there because a larger barnacle, *Balanus*, crowds out the little brown barnacle.

A snail, *Nucella*, likes to eat the larger barnacle *Balanus*, but *Nucella* has more severe exposure limits and can travel only so far up into *Balanus* territory before it risks over-exposure. *Balanus* is safe from this predator as long as it does not dip into *Nucella* territory.

*(continued)*

## Battle on the beach continued

Finally, a low-intertidal species of sea star, *Pisaster*, is a voracious snail predator but doesn't do well when exposed to air for long periods. It eats *Nucella* snails that venture down into the sea star's territory, but *Pisaster* leaves alone snails that keep their proper distance higher in the mid-intertidal.

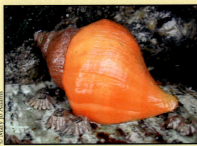

Hundreds of such interactions take place along the intertidal shoreline, where the creatures of each zone live in an arrangement that allows them to meet their needs for growth and reproduction.

© Mary Jo Adams

Atypical orange form of
*Nucella lamellosa*

## Site 3 — CORNET BAY BOAT LAUNCH (Deception Pass State Park)

Lat/Long: 48.4013, -122.6227
West Cornet Bay Rd, Oak Harbor

**Directions:** At traffic light 1 mile S of Deception Pass Bridge, turn E onto Cornet Bay Rd. State park facilities are 1.3 miles on L after private marina.

**Parking:** 110   A Discover Pass is required to park; an additional permit is needed to use boat ramp.

**Adjoining public tideland:** None to west. To east, 2.3 miles around Hoypus Point to southern park boundary. Cornet Bay is a part of Deception Pass State Park, though private tidelands along the southern edge of the bay west of this access interrupt continuous state-owned tidelands.

The park maintains a six-lane, deep-water boat ramp along with a dock, boat pump-out facility, and showers. This is one of only a few boat launches that are available in all tidal conditions on Whidbey Island, but exercise caution as Deception Pass is known for its very strong currents.

To the north is a clear view of lichen-covered bedrock and red-barked madrone trees on the slopes of Goose Rock. Over 1,000 feet of shoreline here has been restored to a more natural condition designed to improve nearshore habitat for salmon and forage fish. Creosote bulkheads and artificial fill were removed, the beach was re-graded to match nearby natural beach slope, and the shore was replanted with native vegetation (see box below).

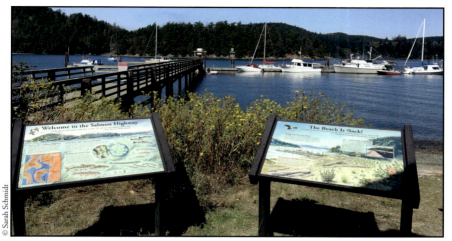

*Dock next to Cornet Bay boat launch*

© Sarah Schmidt

## Shoreline alterations—death by a thousand cuts

In the two centuries since Europeans first sailed into the Salish Sea, they have tried to control nature, changing natural shorelines with a variety of constructions. Materials including stone, concrete, masonry, steel, creosote, and rubber tires have been used to construct bulkheads, groins, pilings, ramps, piers, stairways, and causeways. Often these are poorly planned and unnecessary, designed and built without an understanding of natural processes. These structures can interfere with normal sediment transport, making beaches unusable to forage fish that would otherwise lay thousands of eggs on them. Such structures may block sunlight, hindering or precluding eelgrass growth, and may also leach cancer-causing chemicals into beaches, sediments, and the sea, endangering marine and human life. In addition to habitat destruction, these structures can cause accelerated coastal erosion, thereby damaging the very shoreline they were built to protect.

On Whidbey Island, a restoration project revived 1,600 feet of shoreline and two acres of beach at Cornet Bay in Deception Pass State Park, which had been compromised by creosote armoring and

*(continued)*

## Shoreline alterations continued

and imported fill. Workers removed the armoring and fill, re-graded the beach to match the natural contour, anchored large logs to help establish the driftwood zone, and installed riparian plantings. Within just a few years, forage fish came to spawn, eelgrass meadows flourished, salmon fry migrants found nourishing shelter, and accumulating beach sediments stabilized. This is just one of the successful restoration projects initiated and carried to completion by conservation efforts in Island County to re-establish the natural shorelines that sustain a robust marine habitat.

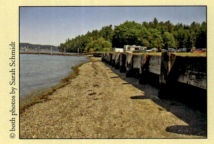
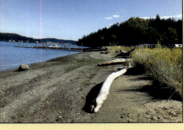

© both photos by Sarah Schmidt

*Cornet Bay 2012 before restoration*    *Cornet Bay 2019 after restoration*

| Site 4 | **HOYPUS POINT** (Deception Pass State Park) |
|---|---|

**HOYPUS POINT** (Deception Pass State Park)
Lat/Long: North entry 48.4112, -122.6074
North entry at end of Cornet Bay Rd;
South entry at end of Ducken Rd, Oak Harbor

**Directions:** *(a) North entry and shore access*–At traffic light 1 mile S of Deception Pass Bridge, turn E onto Cornet Bay Rd and go 1.3 miles to parking area (same as Site 3). Walk the final mile to Hoypus Point, the old launch point of the Deception Pass Ferry before the bridge was built. Access to forest trails from north side is for walkers only. *(b) South entry to trails by Hoypus Hill*– Turn E onto Ducken Rd 0.25 mile S of Cornet Bay Rd. In 0.5 mile, where Monkey Hill Rd curves sharply R, don't turn but continue straight ahead 0.3 mile to parking area. Mountain bikers and horseback riders can access trails here. Adjoins private property; drive slowly.

**Parking:** 110 at end of Cornet Bay Rd; 6 with horse trailers at end of Ducken Rd. A Discover Pass is required for both parking areas.

**Adjoining public tideland:** From Hoypus Point, 1 mile S to park boundary; 1.3 miles NW to Site 3.

(a) From the north parking area at Cornet Bay Rd, walk east on the old road, now closed to vehicles, to reach the shore access at Hoypus Point. Inland hiking trails through the forest reserve pass majestic old-growth Douglas firs six feet in diameter as well as huge western red cedars. At low tide it's a nice beach walk to Hoypus Point.

(b) The Ducken Rd entry provides trail access for horseback riders and mountain bikers. Various trails are restricted to either hikers only; to hikers and horses only; or to hikers, horses, and mountain bikes. Follow signs.

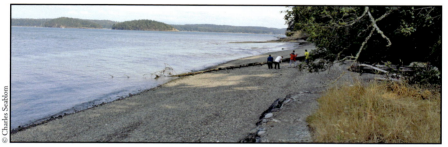

© Charles Seablom

*The Hoypus Point beach provides shade and sun*

## Divers and dabblers dine differently

Each fall, more than two dozen species of wintering ducks and seabirds arrive in our waters. Joining our resident mallards and gadwalls are wigeons, goldeneyes, scoters, loons, and other species.

Watch closely how these species forage for food. Some dabble along the surface, while others dive under the water to feed. The dabblers seek vegetation near the surface, where their horizontally flattened bills aid in filtering surface water as they feed along shallow edges. Dabblers include pintails, wigeons, shovelers, and geese. The category called divers submerge completely underwater, using their feet and occasionally their wings for propulsion, as they forage for swimming fish and for invertebrates along the rocky bottom. These birds have narrow pointed bills, to snatch fish and to poke around looking for invertebrates. Our many divers include buffleheads, goldeneyes, scoters, mergansers, cormorants, grebes, loons, and guillemots.

Watch for dabblers and divers. Knowing these categories will help you find the birds in guides and zero in on identifying unfamiliar species.

# ALA SPIT COUNTY PARK
Lat/Long: 48.3929, -122.5867
5050 Geck Rd, Oak Harbor

**Directions:** Turn E off Hwy 20 at milepost 39.8 (2 miles S of Deception Pass Bridge) onto Troxell Rd. Travel 3.7 miles to Geck Rd on L. Drop down Geck Rd to road end and parking area.

**Parking:** 10-15 🚻 ♨ 🚶 🐟 ⚓ 🚶 ⛺

**Adjoining public tideland:** 1,187 feet of public tidelands.

This 12-acre site includes approximately ¼ mile of public beach, open clamming from May 1 to May 31, and a one-mile round trip walking trail with views of Mount Baker, Mount Erie, and Fidalgo and Hope Islands.

Ala Spit is a narrow ridge of mixed substrate supplied by coastal erosion and transported by nearshore currents. The channel between the spit and Hope Island has provided excellent fishing grounds for recreational anglers.

This is a good place to look at plants found on our shorelines, from eelgrass beds along the beach, to pickleweed on the inland mudflat, to backshore plants (see box pg. 122) along the trail to the end of the spit.

South of the parking area is a Cascadia Marine Trail campsite, permitted only for water access with non-powered boats. Ala Spit is a great launching spot for paddle boarding and kayaking at the spit but avoid pulling boats and boards across sensitive eelgrass habitat.

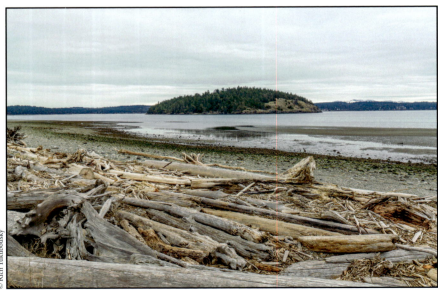

© Rich Yukubousky

*Ala Spit*

## Eelgrass keeps the whole system going

Eelgrass is a nearshore treasure. Entire meadows of this grass-like perennial grow in the shallows off many Island County beaches. It shelters young salmon, forage fish, and invertebrates (creatures with no spinal column) by both buffering the energy of waves and currents and also by providing a safe haven and nursery. Pacific herring lay their eggs on eelgrass. Salmon, in turn, feast on the herring. Anemones, snails, stalked jellyfish, limpets, and nudibranchs anchor themselves to its long, green, ribbon-like leaves. Clams and worms live in the soft sediments surrounding its roots.

Eelgrass grows by spreading its root system under the soft, sandy substrate and by underwater pollination and seed germination. It's one of the very few true plants totally adapted to the marine environment and receives nutrients through its roots and also directly from the water column across its leaf surfaces. Its nutritional value is in the detritus (decaying plant litter) it produces. Like cheese spread on a cracker, eelgrass becomes encrusted with a rich coating of diatoms, bacteria, and protozoa. When the plant dies back or is shredded by wave action, detritus-eating organisms strip the leaf particles of their protein-rich microbial coatings. A single piece of eelgrass detritus can be re-colonized by microbes and passed again and again through the guts of invertebrates.

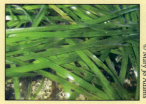

© Mary Jo Adams

Better understanding of the importance of eelgrass is leading to mapping and monitoring of eelgrass meadows and to preserving them through conservation measures.

*Eelgrass*

---

| **Site 6** | **MORAN BEACH** (Powell Rd) |
| | Lat/Long: 48.3729, -122.6657 |
| | 899 Powell Rd, Oak Harbor |

**Directions:** At traffic circle turn W off Hwy 20 onto Banta Rd. Turn N onto Moran Rd, then W onto Powell Rd to road end, approximately 0.8 mile from Hwy 20.

**Parking:** 10-15+ 🚻 ♿ Toilet seasonal.

**Adjoining public tideland:** 100 feet, directly in front of the paved parking lot and road end. Private tidelands to each side are well signed.

This sandy beach offers a sweeping view of the Strait of Juan de Fuca from the San Juan Islands to the Olympics. To the west is the low, flat profile of Smith Island. This location is a great place to relax and enjoy wildlife viewing. As this is a smaller beach surrounded by private property, please be considerate of homeowners and work to keep sand and vegetation clean for marine life. This is a day use only beach; please abide by posted signs.

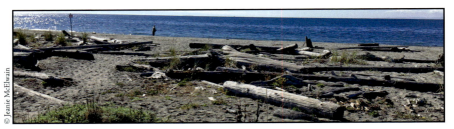

© Jeanie McElwain

*Moran Beach*

## Crustacean molts—the shell game

What looks like a dead crab on the beach may not be what it appears.

If you've ever dined on freshly-cooked crab or shrimp, you know about the rigid outer covering that must be removed before getting to the delicious sweet meat. This outer covering or exoskeleton is secreted by the epidermis and hardens into the animal's shell-like support structure.

As crustaceans grow, every so often they must shed their exoskeleton and replace it with a larger one—a process called molting. As the animal prepares to molt, it secretes a new, soft cuticle under its outer shell. The old shell splits along specific breaking points and the entire animal wriggles out, down to the last tiny claw and even the cuticle covering the eyeball.

Right after molting, while in the soft-shell stage, the animal pumps itself full of water to stretch the new soft cuticle into a larger covering. After the new shell has been hardened with calcium taken up from seawater, the water is pumped out and replaced by animal tissue as the crustacean grows. Young animals molt several times a year; older animals less often, or they may stop molting.

On the beach, molted exoskeletons often are mistaken for dead animals. To find out whether an empty skeleton is a molt or a dead animal, smell it! A molt will have only the fresh smell of the seashore.

<table>
<tr><td>**Site 7**</td><td>## DUGUALLA BAY PRESERVE<br>Lat/Long: 48.3548, -122.5935<br>4021 Dike Rd, Oak Harbor</td></tr>
</table>

**Directions:** Turn E off Hwy 20 onto Frostad Rd. In 0.8 mile turn L onto Dike Rd; at the first turn there is a small parking area.

**Parking:** 8 with additional parking on E side of Dike Rd across from pump station where there is a wide shoulder at the head of the bay.

**Adjoining public tideland:** To north 1.5 miles along Department of Natural Resources Beach 145, below a steep bluff.

With multiple habitats in one place, this is a great place for viewing not only the Cascades to the east, but also the many forms of life close by. At low tides the bay east of the dike becomes a ¼-mile-long mudflat with rich feeding for birds. A large expanse of fresh water inside the dike provides habitat for waterfowl and shorebirds. From the north end of the dike, you can walk the shore along Department of Natural Resources (DNR) Beach 145 below a steep bluff. This site lies under one of the main approaches to Whidbey Island Naval Air Station to the west, so you could be surprised by low-flying aircraft.

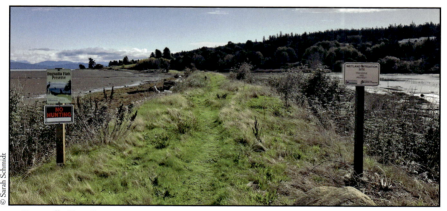

*Dugualla Bay Preserve*

<table>
<tr><td>**Site 8**</td><td>## DUGUALLA STATE PARK<br>Lat/Long: 48.3434, -122.5554 (where the trail ends at the beach)<br>799 E Sleeper Rd, Oak Harbor</td></tr>
</table>

**Directions:** From Hwy 20 turn E onto Sleeper Rd, go 2.6 miles to road end and gate at park boundary.

**Parking:** 10 at park entrance. A Discover Pass is required to park here.

![icons]

**Adjoining public tideland:** 1.25 miles.

This 600-acre park, formerly DNR School Trust Forest land, has over 4 miles of woodland trails. It's a 1½ mile walk to the shore. From the gate, follow the single-lane dirt road to a Y, take right fork in ¼ mile to another Y, take left fork, and in ¼ mile reach end of dirt road. From here a trail winds steeply downhill past some enormous old trees to the beach. The park has nearly 1¼ miles of public shoreline, though at high tides much of the beach is covered by water and isn't walkable. Trail entrance from the beach can be hard to spot so note the location to return to. Sections of this shaded beach provide ideal spawning habitat for forage fish. Day use only. There are no amenities.

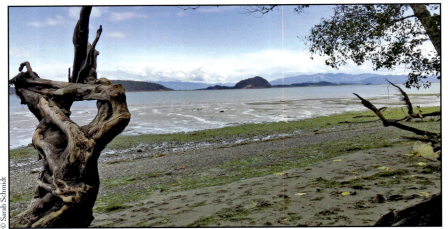

© Sarah Schmidt

*Dugualla State Park*

## Overhanging trees help fish eggs survive

Trees and brush at the base of eroding beach slopes often reach out toward the water at a nearly horizontal angle. This can make it difficult to walk the beach at high tide, tempting landowners to cut the overhanging vegetation. But if left in place, these trees provide priceless shading and cooling of the beach gravels, greatly improving survival of forage fish eggs that would otherwise be killed by harsh midday temperatures. On a sunny day, shoreside cover can keep the beach surface as much as 10° F cooler than a bare beach. Native vegetation on bluff slopes also helps to stabilize the bluff, reducing the threat of landslides.

| Site 9 | **BORGMAN ROAD END** |
|---|---|
| | Lat/Long: 48.3228, -122.5226 |
| | 3092 N Borgman Rd, Oak Harbor |

**Directions: a)** *From N of Oak Harbor,* turn off Hwy 20 onto Fakkema Rd, then S onto Taylor Rd. In 0.8 mile turn E onto Silver Lake Rd, travel 3.5 miles, then go N onto Green Rd for 0.25 mile, then E onto Borgman Rd and down short slope to road end. **b)** *From downtown Oak Harbor,* go E on Pioneer Way, turn L onto Regatta Rd, then E onto Crescent Harbor Rd. In 2 miles turn N onto Taylor Rd and in 0.25 mile E onto Silver Lake Rd. Follow remaining directions above.

**Parking:** 5 ⚓ 🅿

**Adjoining public tideland:** Width of roadway only, approximately 40 feet.

This usually quiet site offers an expansive view of Mount Baker and the Skagit Delta. The frequent buildup of large logs at the road end can make the walk to the beach difficult. When clear and at high tide, it offers access for launching kayak or canoe. The site is surrounded by residential development, so please respect the privacy of those who live there.

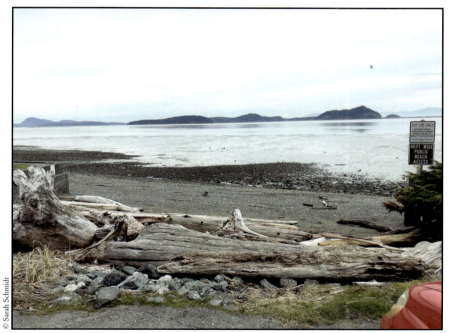

*Borgman Road End*

© Sarah Schmidt

# Whidbey & Camano Islands: In the Salish Sea

When George Vancouver first named Puget Sound in 1792, the area referred to only the Tacoma Narrows, south of Seattle. Over time, the Puget Sound name became popular and included ever-more area, even to waters around the San Juan Islands and southern Georgia Strait in Canada.

Beginning in the 1970s, scientific studies showed that the ecology of the Strait of Georgia, the Strait of Juan de Fuca, and areas called Puget Sound were better understood as a single and integral ecosystem: an inland sea. This ecosystem differs from the ecosystems of the Pacific Ocean west of the Strait of Juan de Fuca as well as the deep and fjord-like channels of the inside passage north of the Strait of Georgia.

This inland sea encompasses 5,500 square miles and opens to the Pacific Ocean through the Strait of Juan de Fuca, a 90-mile long and narrow channel that funnels cold ocean water in and out of the system. Rivers, such as Canada's Fraser River and the Skagit River, feed fresh water and sediment into the Salish Sea, often building deltas in the process. The entire seaway is a complex system including sandy beaches, bluffs, rocky headlands, estuaries, small bays, and canals.

A name was needed to identify this ecosystem, and after much debate, the name Salish Sea, acknowledging the first peoples to live on its shores, began to be accepted, appearing on maps and in studies and books. In 2005, 70 Tribes and First Nations from Washington state and British Columbia collectively formed the Coast Salish Gathering to protect and manage the resources of the Salish Sea.

In 2009 and 2010, the governments of the United States and Canada approved the name Salish Sea as an official designation for these inland, environmentally-linked marine waters of Washington and British Columbia. A celebration by Coast Salish Tribes of Washington State and First Nations of British Columbia was held in July 2010 at the Songhee First Nation in Esquimalt, BC. The event attracted over 2,500 participants who celebrated the Salish Sea name in word, dance, and song.

Nonetheless, change comes slowly, and Salish Sea remains unknown to many people. Because of this, Whidbey and Camano Islands continue to be recognized as islands within Puget Sound as well as within the Salish Sea.

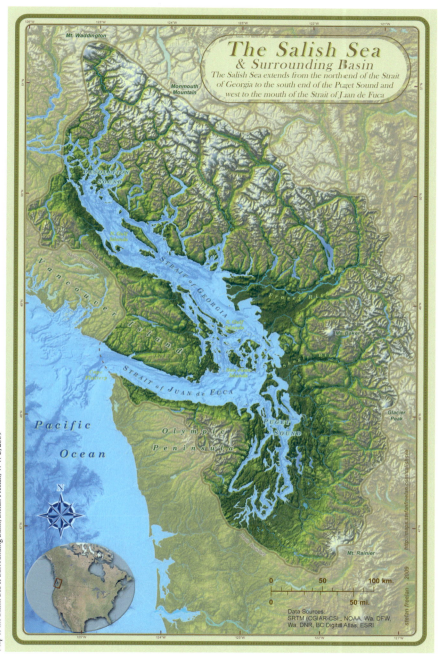

The Salish Sea
& Surrounding Basin

The Salish Sea extends from the north end of the Strait of Georgia to the south end of the Puget Sound and west to the mouth of the Strait of Juan de Fuca

Data Sources:
SRTM (CGIAR-CSI, NOAA, Wa. DFW, Wa. DNR, BC Digital Atlas, ESRI

Map of the Salish Sea & Surrounding Basin, Stefan Freelan, WWU, 2009

The Salish Sea and Surrounding Basin map was produced using a Geographic Information System (GIS) and publicly available spatial datasets for elevation, bathymetry, and hydrology.

# MARINER'S COVE BOAT RAMP
Lat/Long: 48.2898, -122.5179
2200 Mariner Beach Dr, Oak Harbor

**Directions:** From Hwy 20 or Pioneer Way, turn onto Regatta Dr. Turn E onto Crescent Harbor Rd. In 3.5 miles road turns S and becomes Reservation Rd, then in another 1.5 miles turns E and becomes Polnell Rd. After another 2.5 miles, where Polnell Rd becomes Strawberry Point Rd, turn E downhill onto Mariner Beach Dr. Follow 0.4 mi to public access on the L before end of road where you'll find a loop gravel pullout with lawn, bench, and small boat launch.

**Parking:** 8

**Adjoining public tideland:** 245 feet.

Drift log buildup may block the small boat ramp. The view sweeps from Mount Baker to Glacier Peak and the Skagit Delta. Utsalady Point on Camano Island is two miles across the water to the south. The waters along this beach often run muddy, especially after a heavy rainfall, due to sediment flowing from the North Fork of the Skagit River. The Skagit River accounts for roughly 35% of sediment discharge in the Puget Sound lowland. This access has close neighbors and requires special attention and respect for private property.

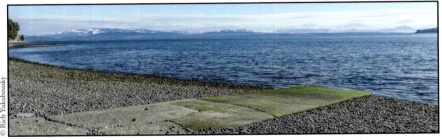

© Rich Yukubousky

*Mariner's Cove boat ramp and beach. Boat ramp is non-commercial only.*

## Seal pups often rest on the beach; please leave them alone

Every year, someone comes upon an adorable seal pup on the beach and thinks it's been abandoned. These well-meaning people have good intentions but do all the wrong things.

Harbor seal birthing season in our region runs from late June through the end of August. Nursing pups stay with their mothers for 4 to 6 weeks and are then weaned to feed and survive on their own.

*(continued)*

## Seal pups continued

Harbor seal pups may haul out in the same place for several days or weeks at a time, and this does not mean they're abandoned. Weaned pups will spend extended hours on shore, resting and regulating their body temperatures. They may be too young to have developed an escape response, so may not flee when approached.

By far the best way to help a pup is to leave it alone. Keep your distance. It's against federal law to disturb any marine mammal or come within 100 yards of its location. Approaching too closely to the pup, pouring water on it, attempting to feed it, or removing it from the beach is unsafe for you and the pup, and it's illegal. In addition, seals and other marine mammals can carry diseases transmissible to humans, pets, and livestock, providing yet another reason to keep people and dogs at least 100 yeards away.

If a pup is on a beach where it may be disturbed, volunteers from the Central Puget Sound Marine Mammal Stranding Network can help keep people away and keep the seal safe. To report a stranded or injured seal pup, or other marine mammal in Island and Skagit counties, call 1-866-ORCANET (866-672-2638). To report harassment of a seal pup or other marine mammal, call the NCAA Enforcement Hotline 1-800-853-1964.

## Site 11 — OAK HARBOR CITY MARINA
Lat/Long: 48.2872, -122.6327
1401 Catalina Dr, Oak Harbor

**Directions:** Located in the City of Oak Harbor. *From the south:* At traffic light where Hwy 20 makes 90° turn to the north, continue straight onto Pioneer Way. *From the north:* At traffic light where Hwy 20 makes 90° turn to the right, turn L onto Pioneer Way. Travel 1.2 miles, turning R into marina on Catalina Dr just before security gate to Navy Seaplane Base. For boat launch, drive past storage sheds and turn R toward water.

**Parking:** 50+ 

**Adjoining public tideland:** Approximately 0.5 mile.

The marina has a very limited beach area to walk, but a paved footpath above the shoreline connects to Sites 12-14. The entire marina is open to the public, including the docks, which have picnic tables at the ends. A play and picnic area is north of the park office. A small park next to the boat ramp at the south end of the property is a great place from which to watch the harbor activity. More information at **ohmarina.org**.

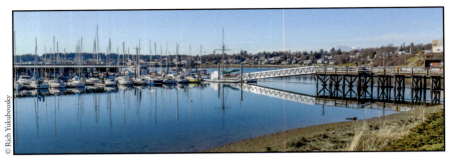

*Oak Harbor City Marina*

| **Site 12** | **PIONEER WAY EAST** |
| | Lat/Long: 48.2895, -122.6387 |
| | 1601 SE Pioneer Way, Oak Harbor |

**Directions:** Located in old downtown Oak Harbor. **a)** *From the south:* At traffic light where Hwy 20 makes 90° turn to the north, continue straight onto Pioneer Way. **b)** *From the north:* At traffic light where Hwy 20 makes 90° turn to the right, turn L onto Pioneer Way. Proceed 0.5 mile past commercial district to waterside parking. Park along the road and access the beach via the stairs.

**Parking:** Along street.

**Adjoining public tideland:** 644 feet opposite Pasek St.

East of the intersection with Bayshore Drive, a sidewalk parallels the shore beside Pioneer Way. Extensive mudflats are exposed at low tide, accessed by stairways that may occasionally be blocked by driftwood. As always, exercise caution walking near exposed mudflats where you could get stuck.

The shorefront has mixed ownership, with some sections belonging to homeowners across the street. Please respect any stairs posted private.

This waterfront was being damaged by *Spartina*, an invasive non-native grass (see box on next page). Community volunteers worked with the county Noxious Weed Control Board, and in 2019 the area had been clear of *Spartina* for three years.

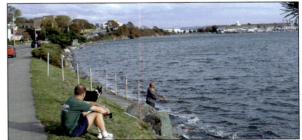

*Pioneer Way East*

## *Spartina* cordgrass, a destructive shoreline invader

Common cordgrass, or *Spartina angelica*, is a halophyte, a terrestrial plant adapted to grow in salt water. In the 1960s, farmers planted what they believed to be sterile hybrid seed along tidelands in an attempt to increase the amount of land where cattle could graze. Unfortunately, the seed was not sterile and spread, eventually infesting thousands of acres.

*Spartina* utterly transforms the ecosystem, displacing native vegetation and raising the elevation of the area where it establishes. Its dense root system traps sediment, turning eelgrass beds and mudflats into grass-choked marshes. It's a grave threat to native fish, shellfish, and migrating shorebirds. Once established, it's very difficult to remove.

In partnership with community volunteers, Island County has worked for decades to eradicate *Spartina* from our tidelands. In 2019, less than one solid acre of *Spartina* plants was recorded along all of the county's shorelines, lagoons, and bays – down from 450 solid acres in 1997. Successful removal of plants along Oak Harbor's Bayshore Drive waterfront has resulted in no new plants there since 2016. However, healthy populations still propagate at a few Island County sites to serve as seed and root distributors, which can re-establish plants quickly along shorelines.

To report *Spartina* cordgrass growing in tidelands, contact the county Noxious Weed Coordinator; search online for Island County Noxious Weed Control Board.

| Site 13 | **FLINTSTONE PARK**<br>Lat/Long: 48.2868, -122.6472<br>1402 SE Dock St, Oak Harbor |

**Directions:** Located in the City of Oak Harbor. **a)** *From the south:* At traffic light where Hwy 20 makes 90° turn to the north, continue straight onto Pioneer Way. **b)** *From the north:* At traffic light where Hwy 20 makes 90° turn to the right, turn L onto Pioneer Way. At next traffic light, turn S onto SE City Beach St, then E on Bayshore Dr. The Park is on S side after Dock St.

**Parking:** 13+ in park plus parking along street.

🚻 🚽 ⛩ ⛺ 🥾 🛩 🛶 🚩 🚶 🏕 Dock is seasonal.

**Adjoining public tideland:** 415 feet.

This quiet park and mini-harbor provides an excellent view of the Oak Harbor Marina. Sit on the sandy beach with the ducks and watch the boat traffic in the harbor. Seasonal docks provide platforms for fishing and day-use moorage for shallow-draft boats. Watch out for tides that can leave a boat stranded and exposed mudflats that can leave a beach walker stuck and sinking. A waterfront trail can also be accessed from this site. Stop by the cement Flintstone car for a unique reminder of your trip.

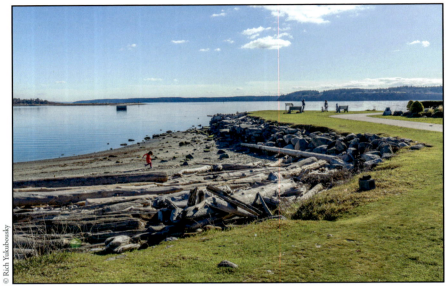

© Rich Yukubousky

*Flintstone Park*

## Before the bridge

Just one of many early ferry services in Island County was the Oak Harbor–Utsalady ferry that ran from 1925-1935, linking the county's two populated islands much more directly than today's three-county drive. The ferry *Acorn* was owned by the husband-wife team of Agaton and Berte Olson, who also operated the Deception Pass Ferry. Berte Olson was the stuff of legends, becoming Washington's first licensed female ferry boat skipper. From the arrival of the first white settlers in the 1850s until completion of the Deception Pass Bridge in 1935, transportation in Island County was focused on the water. Early maritime transportation took place in sailing ships and canoes with hired crews of Indians to paddle them, but during the

*(continued)*

## Before the bridge continued

Mosquito Fleet era it shifted to stern-wheelers, side-wheelers, and propeller-driven ships. Many early communities, such as Langley, did a thriving business supplying wood to keep the boilers going on these steam-powered vessels.

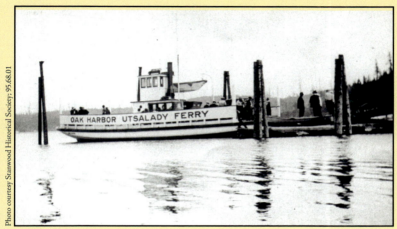

Photo courtesy Stanwood Historical Society; 95.68.01

*The* Acorn, *circa 1925.*

**Site 14**

## WINDJAMMER PARK (aka City Beach)
Lat/Long: at boat ramp 48.2835, -122.6562
End of SE City Beach St (east entrance)
1600 SW Beeksma Dr (west entrance), Oak Harbor

**Directions:** Located in the City of Oak Harbor. **East entrance**—*a) From the south,* at traffic light where Hwy 20 makes 90° turn to the L, continue straight onto Pioneer Way; or *b) From the north,* at traffic light where Hwy 20 makes 90° turn to the R, turn L onto Pioneer Way. At next traffic light, turn R onto SE City Beach St and continue straight into parking area close to playground, splash park, swimming lagoon, and waterside picnic tables. **West entrance**—*a) From the south,* at traffic light where Hwy 20 makes 90° turn to the L, turn R onto Beeksma Dr; or *b) From the north,* at traffic light where Hwy 20 makes 90° turn to the R, continue straight onto Beeksma Dr. This provides access to a tide-dependent single-lane boat ramp and a large parking lot

**Parking:** (East) At the end of City Beach St, 36 spaces. (West) Off Beeksma Dr, 25 spaces near shoreline and boat ramp, plus 135 spaces inland.

**Adjoining public tideland:** 2,100 feet

This popular family park has a splash park, a swimming lagoon, two playgrounds for small children, two large picnic shelters with reservable kitchens, Little League and practice fields, and two basketball courts. The narrow boat ramp is tide limited; consider the deep-water ramp at Site 11.

A paved footpath follows the shoreline, stretching 1½ miles from Beeksma Dr to the marina. The view spans past the mouth of Penn Cove down Saratoga Passage, and east above the masts of moored boats to the distant snow-capped Cascades. West from Beeksma Dr, a graveled trail crosses Freund's Marsh to a parking area for 6-8 cars at Scenic Heights Rd. Windjammer Park has something for everyone and is very popular. With that in mind, we encourage you to enjoy the beach responsibly by packing out everything you bring, disposing of refuse appropriately, and maintaining a safe distance from marine birds and mammals.

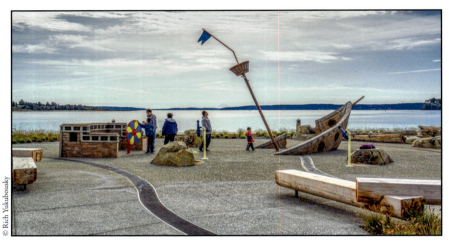

*Shipwreck Shores Splash Park at Windjammer Park*

| Site 15 | **ROCKY POINT PICNIC AREA** (U.S. Navy restricted) |
| | Rocky Point Road, Oak Harbor |

**Directions:** From Hwy 20, W onto Ault Field Rd. In 2 miles continue W on Clover Valley Rd (straight through traffic circle). After 0.8 mile where road curves L, turn R onto Navy land toward Rocky Point Picnic Area. Drive all the way to end, beyond pavement down to graveled beach parking area.

**Parking:** 20+

**Adjoining public tideland:** South 0.5 mile to Joseph Whidbey State Park.

This sand beach, property of the U.S. Navy, is open to anyone with a Department of Defense U.S. Uniformed Services ID card. Others wanting permission to walk the beach may send a letter to the Base Commanding Officer. The beach meets Joseph Whidbey State Park to the south. There is a live firing range between, so pay attention to warning flags and signs. This location offers a beautiful stretch of sandy beach with expansive views to the Strait of Juan de Fuca and the San Juan Islands.

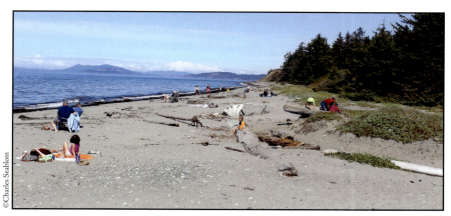

*Rocky Point Picnic Area (U.S. Navy)*

## Site 16 — JOSEPH WHIDBEY STATE PARK

Lat/Long (WA Water Trails campsite) 48.3089, -122.7144; [beach at parking area (1)] 48.3079, -122.7163
2699 W Beach Rd, Oak Harbor

**Directions:** *a) From Oak Harbor* turn W off Hwy 20 onto Swantown Rd. Travel 3 miles to stop sign at T intersection with Crosby Rd. The state park entrance is opposite on N side of Crosby. There are two other parking areas with no facilities: (1) turn L onto Crosby Rd to public beach access at bottom of hill immediately N of first residence where West Beach Rd turns S; or (2) turn R onto Crosby Rd for 0.75 mile; Crosby curves L, then R; entrance to unpaved parking area is on NW side on second curve. *b) From the south,* turn W off Hwy 20 onto Libbey Rd, then N onto West Beach Rd for 5.7 miles to Joseph Whidbey State Park.

**Parking: 25+** A Discover Pass is required to park within park boundaries.

Toilet, ADA accessible, is seasonal.

**Adjoining public tideland:** Northward 0.6 mile to park boundary. Beyond is the beach adjoining Rocky Point Picnic Area (Site 15).

Ocean vistas, picnic sites, fields for playing, and several miles of walking on beach, field, and forest are found at 112-acre Joseph Whidbey State Park, which is administered by Fort Ebey State Park. A mile-long loop trail through forest and field can be reached from the main parking area or parking area 2 on Crosby Rd. The low profile of Smith and Minor islands, which are joined at low tide, can be seen four miles offshore in the Strait of Juan de Fuca.

Park facilities are closed Oct. 1-Mar. 31, but the park is open for day use; year-round parking is available at the two alternate parking areas. A Washington Water Trails water-access-only campsite, located at the northernmost corner of the lower lawn (the only camping allowed in the park), may be accessed by human or wind-powered watercraft only; check with the park for camping fees.

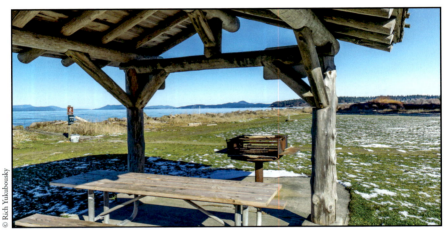

*Joseph Whidbey State Park*

| Site 17 | **WEST BEACH VISTA** (aka Sunset Beach) |
|---------|-----------------------------------------|
|         | Lat/Long: 48.2982, -122.7251 |
|         | 2407 West Beach Rd, Oak Harbor |

**Directions:** Follow directions for Site 16. Continue 0.8 miles S on West Beach Rd, paralleling the shore between a row of residences to W and Swan Lake to E. South of the houses, park on W side of road uphill at fenced overlook.

**Parking:** 10 🛩 🚶 🎣 🚶 🏕

**Adjoining public tideland:** To south approximately 2 miles.

This unimproved site under Island County ownership is a popular place to view Salish Sea sunsets, the San Juan Islands, and the Olympic Mountains. It's also a good place to witness the limits of human efforts to control nature. A huge concrete seawall lies in ruins here, left from a failed attempt to create beachfront property along a dynamic (moving) shoreline.

<table>
<tr><td>**Site 18**</td><td># HASTIE LAKE COUNTY PARK<br>Lat/Long: 48.2644, -122.7484<br>2434 Hastie Lake Road, Oak Harbor</td></tr>
</table>

**Directions:** *a) From the north,* turn W off Hwy 20 onto Hastie Lake Rd. Follow Hastie Lake Rd 2.5 miles across West Beach Rd to road end and County Park. *b) From the south,* turn W off Hwy 20 onto Libbey Rd, then N onto West Beach Rd for 2.25 miles to Hastie Lake Rd, turn L into parking lot.

**Parking:** 10 ⬛ 🚶 🛥 🏕

**Adjoining public tideland:** Below meander line (see pg. 3), 700 feet to north and 2.4 miles south to Site 20. At this site, the meander line is somewhat marked on the low tide between the sandy beach and the cobblestones. Walk only on the cobblestoned area to access public tidelands as you move north and south.

Enjoy a view of the Olympic Mountains, Vancouver Island, and the San Juan Islands. An ADA parking site adjoins a bench next to the boat ramp. The boat ramp is limited to use during conditions of slack water and no winds. Walk the beach southward below towering bluffs, but be cautious about tide levels. In places, waves at high tide reach the foot of the bluffs; don't get trapped. Caution should also be exercised around the bluffs themselves as landslides could make this dangerous. This access has close neighbors. Please pay attention and respect private property.

Much of the glacial material of this beach originated from igneous, metamorphic, and sedimentary rocks of the coastal mountains in British Columbia. The larger rocks provide a measure of erosion protection as they dissipate wave energy.

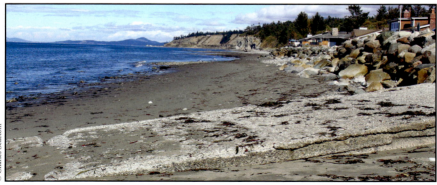

*Hastie Lake County Park*

# The Coast Salish peoples

Millennia before Europeans arrived in their tall ships, Coast Salish peoples fished, hunted, gathered shellfish and berries, built plank houses, and traveled by canoe among permanent and seasonal villages throughout the Pacific Northwest, including British Columbia. Clovis spear points found at prehistoric sites on Penn Cove were used in hunting the Columbian mammoth, which roamed Whidbey Island after the last ice age. This indicates humans have inhabited central Whidbey for over 10,000 years. Thirty-four archeological sites have been found around Penn Cove alone, including three permanent Salish villages.

Families intermarried over a large area and participated in a potlatch economic system where resources were regularly shared. On Ebey's Prairie on Whidbey Island, they encouraged the root crops bracken fern and camas through selective burning. They trapped salmon in nearby rivers, harvested shellfish from Penn Cove, hunted game, and harvested wild potatoes, berries, and other plants. The area's bountiful resources produced a natural surplus of many foods, which enabled the Salish to develop a social organization that went beyond foraging to accommodate specialists. This surplus also allowed for the large populations and permanent village sites found in most of the sheltered coves on the lee side of the islands. Puget Sound Coast Salish used a distinctive weaving style that included the use of dog fur, mountain goat wool, and plant fibers. They are also known for their carving and sophisticated basket weaving.

European diseases took a staggering toll after first contact. In 1855, Puget Sound Coast Salish leaders signed the Treaty of Point Elliot and ceded their lands. Laws were passed making Coast Salish traditional economic and religious practices illegal, and speaking Coast Salish languages was forbidden in schools. Other attempts at cultural assimilation occurred also. Today many Coast Salish people are reclaiming their traditional heritage while living in the modern world and making use of modern resources. The Penn Cove Water Festival, with its popular Native canoe races, celebrates and honors this long heritage. The Hibulb Cultural Center and Natural History Preserve (hibulbculturalcenter.org) in Tulalip (on the mainland due east of Langley), offers hours of exploration into the culture of the Coast Salish peoples.

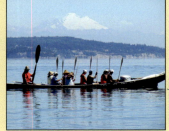

© Sally Slotterback

| Site 19 | **MONROE LANDING** |
|---------|---------------------|

Lat/Long: 48.2402, -122.6806
512 Scenic Heights Rd, Oak Harbor

**Directions:** *a) From the north*, turn S off Hwy 20 onto Monroe Landing Rd. Follow this road almost 2 miles to road end. The park is directly in front of you, with a gravel lot for boat trailers across the street. *b) From the south*, turn E off Hwy 20 onto Arnold Rd to Monroe Landing Rd, then turn R to the park.

**Parking:** 8 on each side of Penn Cove Rd.

Toilet seasonal.

**Adjoining public tideland:** 0.5 mile to east, none to west.

Monroe Landing, a ¼-acre park located on Penn Cove across from the town of Coupeville, offers a striking view of the Olympic mountain range. A portable toilet is on site June 1 to September 1. At low tide on this sandy/cobble beach, you can easily locate the burrows of ghost shrimp (see box pgs. 91-92). Private beach is to the west. As early as 1300 near this site, the Skwdab, a subgroup of the Skagit, had a permanent settlement with a longhouse built on a 4,000-year-old midden. Skwdab territory included Oak Harbor and Dugualla Bay, and until the early 1900s, surrounding tribes traveled by canoe to this last of the Whidbey Island longhouses for potlatch ceremonies.

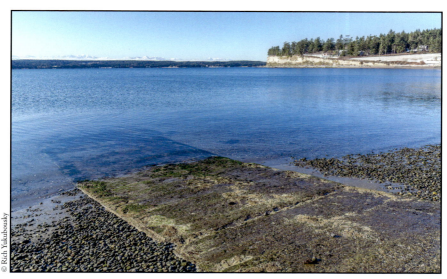

© Rich Yukubousky

*Monroe Landing*

# Sea star wasting disease

Since first detected in 2013, sea stars along the Pacific coast of North America have been dying by the millions from the syndrome "sea star wasting disease." Though sea star die-off had occurred before, it wasn't as widely spread or quickly devastating. Currently, entire sea star populations in the Salish Sea are being eradicated, with a 95% mortality rate. Sea stars first show symptoms of the disease with lesions and withering legs, then advance to tissue decay and loss of legs completely, and then to death with body desiccation within three days. Occurrence is sporadic but leads to mass mortality for the affected sea stars. Scientists are still unsure of the cause as they study different pathogens; the impact of climate change is likely a contributing factor.

Two of the sea stars significantly affected in the Salish Sea are the ochre or purple sea star (*Pisaster ochraceus*) and the sunflower sea star (*Pycnopodia helianthoides*). These are designated as keystone species because they have an exceptionally broad influence on all other species in the ecosystem, and their disappearance drastically reduces the balance of marine life diversity. For example, the sunflower star's primary diet is sea urchin, whose primary diet is kelp. Without the sunflower star, the increasing sea urchin population may destroy the kelp, which provides vital shelter and habitat for juvenile fish and countless invertebrates, filters sunlight for underwater marine life, and provides oxygen for the earth.

Recent findings show that some sea stars are beginning to make a recovery via genetic mutation. Scientists are working to understand this genetic shift and how it may contribute to new sea star populations in the future. It's important that humans don't inadvertently spread wasting disease from one population to another. Sick sea stars should not be touched. Reasonable precautions to prevent the spread of the disease are advised by researchers at the University of California at Santa Cruz at **seastarwasting. org.** These include brushing or spraying footwear with freshwater to remove trapped material and then spraying with dilute bleach before moving between sites. Search "disinfection bleach" for dilution formula. Replace bleach after three months because it degrades.

| Site 20 | **LIBBEY BEACH PARK** |
|---------|------------------------|
|         | Lat/Long: 48.2321, -122.7668 |
|         | 2750 Libbey Road, Oak Harbor |

**Directions:** Turn W off Hwy 20 onto Libbey Rd (6.5 miles S of Oak Harbor) and follow 1.2 miles to road end. This area is also known as Partridge Point.

**Parking:** 10 ⬛ ⛩ ◈ ⛵ 🚶 ➤ 🏛 Toilet seasonal.

**Adjoining public tideland:** 5 miles to north and 8 miles south to Fort Casey. Tidelands, extending to Hastie Lake (Site 18) to the north are from the meander line to extreme low tide. Tidelands to the south are from ordinary high water to extreme low tide.

With 13 miles of beach to walk, keep track of time and tides as listed for Partridge Point. A high tide could leave you stranded, wet, or hanging from the bluff. This three-acre park offers expansive views of Strait of Juan de Fuca, Olympic Mountains, Vancouver Island, and San Juan Islands. The Smith and Minor Islands Aquatic Reserve offshore contains the largest kelp forest in Washington State (see box below).

Please respect neighboring private property. Beach access is via concrete steps and is tide dependent, especially to the north. Eroding bluffs along this stretch of west Whidbey provide constant nourishment for the beaches. The beach composition is constantly changing and can include any variety of sand, pebble, cobble, boulders, driftwood and logs, and seaweed. This is a great place for wildlife viewing including winter birding. The Fort Ebey State Park beach access point can be reached via the beach by walking about ½ mile south.

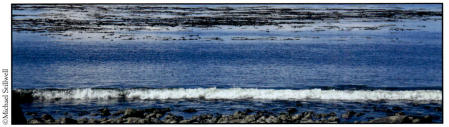

©Michael Stillwell

*Libbey Beach Park*

### Forest of the seas—phytoplankton and seaweeds

A secret world lies just beneath the cold waters of the Pacific Northwest—a smorgasbord of seaweeds growing in layers much like a terrestrial forest of trees, shrubs, and ground covers. Moreover, the entire marine forest is bathed seasonally in a rich soup of single-celled algae called phytoplankton. Each layer of the marine forest has its own complement of fish and invertebrate species.

**The forest canopy:** Large, fast-growing kelps form the tree or canopy layer. *Nereocystis*, commonly known as bull kelp, can grow up to five inches in one day and reach heights of over 30 feet in one growing season.

*(continued)*

## Forest of the Seas continued

**The shrub layer:** Below the kelps are shorter multi-branching foliose and filamentous seaweeds.

**The marine ground covers:** Below the shrubs are the marine ground covers—seaweeds that form carpet-like coverings or thin crusts over rocks.

Like their terrestrial counterparts, seaweeds and single-celled phytoplankton form the base of the Earth's food web. They use chlorophyll and other accessory pigments to harness the sun's energy and convert carbon dioxide and water into sugar molecules. Phytoplankton is found throughout the world's oceans suspended in the water column. Seaweeds attach themselves to rocks and most are restricted to the shallow depths of shoreline that meet their sunlight requirements for growth.

Seaweeds don't have roots or nutrient transport systems like eelgrass and other true plants. They attach themselves to rocks with holdfasts and use their suspended blades to extract nutrients directly from the water column. Like eelgrass, the main food benefit from seaweeds is in the detritus, pieces of dead or dying tissue encrusted with protein-rich mats of microbes, which are consumed by detritus eaters.

Phytoplankton and seaweeds grow rapidly starting in spring (an event referred to as the spring bloom), then die back during fall and winter when there are fewer hours of daylight. Some seaweeds are perennials, surviving more than two years. Others are annuals, renewing themselves each spring.

Phytoplankton and seaweed blooms can also be destructive to marine habitats, smothering invertebrates and other seaweeds and depleting oxygen from the water as they decay. Harmful algal blooms are being reported more frequently around the world; pollution from inadequately treated sewage, agricultural run-off, erosion, and waste from animals—including pets—seems to be a major source of the excess nutrients that cause such blooms.

PLEASE NOTE: THERE ARE LEGAL RESTRICTIONS ON SEAWEED HARVESTING. SEARCH ONLINE FOR *WADNR* SEAWEED HARVEST TO LEARN HOW TO HARVEST SEAWEED LEGALLY.

---

| Site 21 | **FORT EBEY STATE PARK** |
|---------|--------------------------|
| | Lat/Long: WA Water Trails campsite 48.2269, -122.7694 |
| | 400 Hill Valley Drive, Coupeville |

**Directions:** Turn W off Hwy 20 onto Libbey Rd (6.5 miles S of Oak Harbor). Follow Libbey Rd 0.75 mile and turn S onto Hill Valley Dr. Follow 0.75 mile to state park entrance. For beach access, turn R to parking for beach and lake trails 0.5 mile beyond entry booth.

**Parking:** Parking is plentiful. A Discover Pass is required to park here.

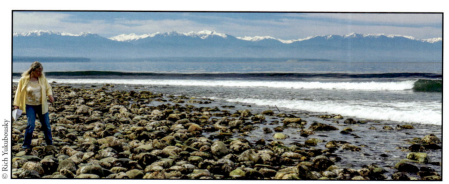

**Adjoining public tideland:** 5.5 miles to north and 7.5 miles south to Fort Casey

The 650-acre park, with three miles of saltwater shoreline on the Strait of Juan de Fuca, is open year-round for day use and May through October for camping. Fort Ebey was constructed in 1942 for coastal defense.

Adjoining the park to the east is an area known for its kettles, large depressions in the earth left as the last glaciers receded. The park and surrounding area feature more than 30 miles of trails for hiking and mountain biking. Horseback riding is allowed on those trails in the kettles area that are not on state park land. Visitors may also explore concrete bunkers and gun batteries, surf, paraglide, or fish for smallmouth bass in Lake Pondilla.

The beach can be accessed at the north end of the park by turning right from the entrance booth to the Beach Parking Lot and the restroom. There are expansive views of the Smith and Minor Islands Aquatic Reserve, Strait of Juan de Fuca, and Olympic Mountains.

You can walk along the beach as far as Fort Casey, about seven miles. Check tides before departing, as high tides can trap you between water and bluff. The beach composition is constantly changing and can include any variety of sand, pebble, cobble, boulders, driftwood, logs, and seaweed. This area, also known as Point Partridge, is a great place for wildlife viewing, including winter birding. There are many marine lookout points along the Bluff Trail.

A single Washington Water Trails campsite, located at the south end of the day-use area near the north beach parking lot, is only for people arriving in non-motorized watercraft.

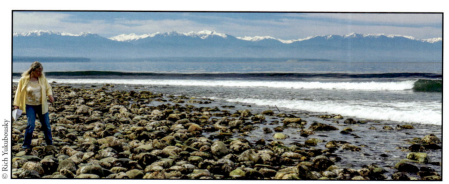

© Rich Yukubousky

*Fort Ebey State Park*

# Birds of the beach

Select any beach around Island County and you may see any of 70 species of birds as you stroll.

The most common will likely be gulls, perched on pilings, standing on mudflats, or floating on the bay. If you see a gull standing in shallow water, watch closely and you may observe it treading the sand to stir up invertebrates for lunch.

A family of crows might fly past or call from overhanging trees. A bald eagle could be perched high on a snag or sitting right on the beach. Gulls, crows, and eagles all scavenge tidbits washed in by the last high tide. Both gulls and crows carry shellfish into the air, then drop them onto rocks or pavement to crack the shells and reach the meat inside.

A group of killdeer might scamper along the sandy beach. If you approach too closely they'll voice a warning. Above them, a belted king-fisher may fire its loud rattling call as it flies up and down the beach. In winter watch for flocks of sanderlings, small shorebirds with gray back, white belly and coal black legs, eyes and bill; they chase waves on sandy beaches in a blur of running feet. Stand still and they may pass close by you.

Out on the water, especially in winter, you can see groups of ducks and seabirds. These could be scoters, buffleheads, goldeneyes, mergansers, and grebes. You might see a black and white loon swimming along, then diving underwater to seek prey.

For more on Puget Sound birds, see birdweb.org.

## Site 22

## GRASSER'S LAGOON
Lat/Long: 48.2340, -122.7316
25741 Hwy 20, Coupeville

**Directions:** On S side of Hwy 20 at the NW corner of Penn Cove, 100 ft W of Zylstra Rd and 0.25 mile E of Madrona Way, turn into U-shaped gravel pullout.

**Parking:** 10-15 A Discover Pass or Washington Vehicle Use Permit (from WDFW) is required to park here. Toilet is seasonal.

**Adjoining public tideland:** To west and south, 0.5 mile.

The mudflats south of the lagoon are popular with clam diggers during low tides. For information on shellfish harvesting rules and seasons, search online for WDFW shellfishing regulations. Bald eagles, kingfishers, seabirds, shorebirds, and waterfowl frequent the area, particularly between October and April. Marine mammals such as harbor seals may be spotted.

## Yes, we have gulls, but no seagulls

Have you ever looked for seagull in the index of a birding guide? It's not listed. That's because these birds are more correctly called gulls, with many species, some of which are found far from the sea.

The most common gull in the Puget Sound lowlands is the glaucous-winged gull (glaucous means gray). Glaucous-winged gulls (most of which, in our region, are actually a hybrid of glaucous-winged and western gulls) have gray wings all the way down to and including their wing tips.

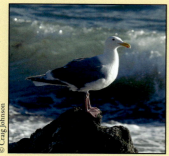
© Craig Johnson

*Glaucous-winged gull*

Through the year, 12 other species of gulls wander into our area. Summer and fall bring large numbers of Bonaparte's gulls, mew gulls, California gulls, and ring-billed gulls, but still well over 70% of all the gulls you see following the ferryboats, scavenging for food, or just standing around are glaucous-winged (hybrid) gulls.

## Site 23 | MUELLER PARK
Lat/Long: 48.2242, -122.7307
Between 2118 and 2110 Madrona Way, Coupeville

**Directions:** From Hwy 20 turn S onto Madrona Way along W end of Penn Cove. Go 0.8 mile to the access, a U-shaped gravel pullout on the E side of Madrona Way about 0.1 mile N of Captain Whidbey Inn. Note the WDFW sign.

**Parking:** 6-8 A Discover Pass or Washington Vehicle Use Permit (from WDFW) is required to park here.

**Adjoining public tideland:** North for about 2,000 feet and south about 0.5 mile around Captain Whidbey Inn.

This beach has been stocked with shellfish by WDFW. Much of the beach surrounds the Captain Whidbey Inn complex. Please respect the privacy of the hotel guests. Be aware of signs indicating shellfish seasons or closures due to shellfish illness.

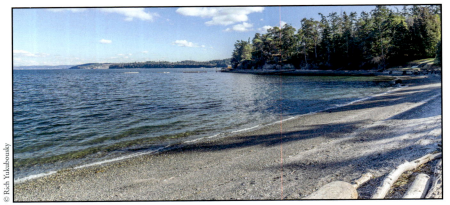

*Mueller Park*

## Penn Cove mussel rafts

Many visitors to the Coupeville area are puzzled by dozens of small rafts anchored in neat rows along the south shore of Penn Cove. These are part of a major aquaculture farm, Penn Cove Shellfish, LLC. Lines are suspended from the rafts, and mussels grow on these lines until they are hoisted from the water and the mussels harvested. Thanks to an accident of geography, Penn Cove serves as a nutrient trap for outflows from the Skagit and Stillaguamish rivers. The influx of fresh water, combined with sunshine from the rain-shadow effect of the Olympic Mountains, fills Penn Cove with a plankton soup ideal for growing mussels. Penn Cove Shellfish also wet-stores and distributes oysters and clams, but over the course of several decades has really made its name known worldwide for mussels.

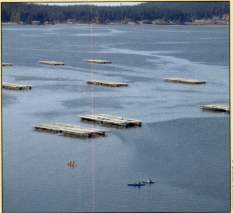

## Site 24 — COUPEVILLE TOWN PARK
### Corner of Coveland St and Coburn, Coupeville

**Directions:** Located in Coupeville uphill from the wharf. From Hwy 20, turn N onto Main St, and in 0.5 mile turn W with the main route onto Coveland St. After crossing Alexander, the road goes uphill; where it splits, the park entrance driveway is on the R.

**Parking:** 16 🚻 🅿️ ⛱ 🏠 🔪 🐚 🏃

**Adjoining public tideland:** To east 0.5 mile.

The park offers broad grassy lawns, a children's play area, picnic facilities, and a gazebo where public events are held. A kiosk holds an enormous slice of a 700-year-old Douglas fir, which was a sapling about 200 years before Columbus arrived in the Americas. From the north side, a dirt trail descends in switchbacks down the bluff to the beach. When beach walking, be aware that waves reach the base of the bluff at high tides. From the east end of the parking lot, a land trail leads along the bluff to the Coupeville wharf, making a nice loop.

## Site 25 — COUPEVILLE WHARF & BEACH ACCESSES
### Lat/Long: 48.2227, -122.6878
### Corner of Front and Alexander Sts, Coupeville

**Directions:** Located on the Coupeville waterfront. From Hwy 20, turn N onto Main St and W onto Coveland St. In 2 blocks, turn N onto Alexander St, go 1 block to wharf.

**Parking:** Parking is along adjoining streets, and in the town lot uphill on Alexander St, near the library. Wharf is wheelchair-accessible.

🚻 🅿️ ⛱ 🐚 🛶 🏃 🚤

**Adjoining public tideland:** 0.5 mile.

A 500-foot walkway leads to the wharf building and dock facilities, owned and operated by the Port of Coupeville. The wharf building holds an extensive display of the interconnectedness of marine life and human activity, past and present, in Penn Cove: An eelgrass habitat mural; skeletons of a gray whale, Dall's porpoise, and Steller's sea lion suspended from the ceiling; geologic and Coast Salish history; orca activity; impacts of pollution; and a selection of videos to captivate the attention of both children and adults.

Once the heart of Whidbey Island, Coupeville was served by Mosquito Fleet steamboat service from the 1890s to 1937, connecting it with Seattle, Everett, and many small towns (see box pg. 120). During lower tides, abundant sea life may be visible from the wharf, including barnacles, mussels, jellyfish, sea stars, and fish.

The shoreline can be accessed by two stairways, one at the foot of the wharf and another two blocks E at the foot of Main St. Hand-carry boats can be launched from the dock attached to the wharf, but this requires carrying them the length of the dock and down a narrow ramp. Use the boat launch at Site 26 unless the tide is too low.

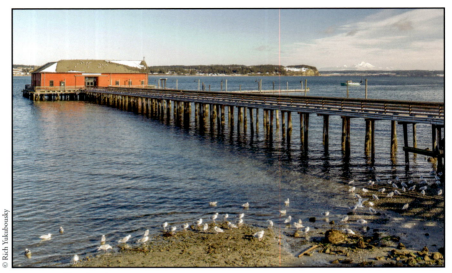

© Rich Yukubousky

*Coupeville wharf*

### What is an invasive species?

An invasive species is a plant or animal that is not native to a region and damages the balance within the native ecosystem, causing societal, economic, and environmental harm. According to the International Union for Conservation of Nature, "Invasive alien species are the second most significant threat to biodiversity, after habitat loss. In their new ecosystems, (they) become predators, competitors, parasites, hybridizers, and diseases of our native and domesticated plants and animals."

On Whidbey and Camano Islands, invasive species include European green crab (next page), Atlantic salmon, *Spartina* cordgrass (see box pg. 39), Scotch broom, tansy ragwort, and five thistle species, to cite just a few. For information on identification and control of noxious weeds: **whidbeycd.org /weed-bulletin.**

## The invasive green crab

The European green crab (native to the Atlantic Ocean shores of Europe and Africa) has recently found its way into the Salish Sea and to the shores of Whidbey Island. This invasive species is a voracious predator and potentially out-competes native crabs for food and habitat. The green crab also decimates native clams and oysters, its primary prey. This threatens the ecological balance of marine life native to the Salish Sea region.

You can be "the eyes on the beach" by identifying and reporting this invasive crab. It's best identified by the set of five saw-toothed spines on the front end of the carapace (shell) on either side of its eyes. Its color is not necessarily green and can vary, depending on its age and its surroundings. If you believe you've found and identified a green crab, leave it where you found it and call WDFW at 1-888-933-9247 or email photos and details to **crabteam@uw.edu**. (Leave the crab on the beach because it is illegal to possess a live green crab without a permit.) Additional information on this invasive species is available online by searching invasive green crab.

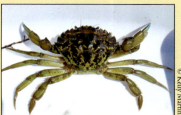

© Kelly Martin

---

**Site 26** | **CAPTAIN COUPE PARK**
Lat/Long: 48.2205, -122.6784
600 NE 9th St, Coupeville

**Directions:** Located in Coupeville. From Hwy 20, turn N onto Main St and E onto 9th St. Go six blocks, turn L into park immediately past sewage treatment plant.

**Parking:** 10-12 as a combination of car and trailer spots.

**Adjoining public tideland:** 1.6 miles east to Long Point.

In good conditions and sufficiently high tides, this is a good boat launch site. Boat launching and retrieval can be a problem due to strong northwest winds. At low tide the dock sits atop mudflats. The tidelands here are typical for inland waters that have low wave impacts. Mudflats are filled with clams and other burrowing organisms, and surface substrates support barnacle and mussel communities. The area is known for spawning smelt and supports limited eelgrass beds. This beach is within the closure area for a sewage treatment plant outfall and is closed year-round for recreational shellfish harvesting. A roadside pedestrian trail running from Captain Coupe Park to the Front Street commercial district offers views and resting benches.

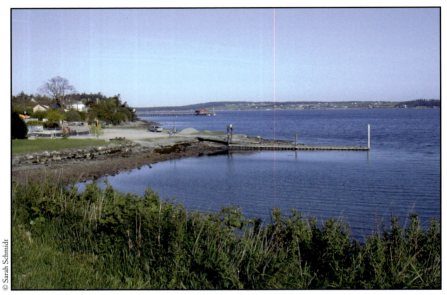

Captain Coupe Park

## Salmon cruise the eelgrass highway

Island County sits at the center of the Salish Sea, on the migration corridors used by salmon from nearly all of its major river systems. The many pocket estuaries and eelgrass beds on both sides of the islands provide critical shelter and refuge from predators as well as high-energy marine environments.

Migrating salmon feed on herring, which lay their eggs directly on the eelgrass. Salmon also consume surf smelt and sand lance, which spawn on the gravels of Island County's many healthy beaches.

Because eelgrass beds and healthy beaches are vitally important to the entire marine food chain, Sound Water Stewards, Island County Marine Resources Committee (MRC), and others monitor eelgrass health and also foster public understanding of how we can help preserve and protect these precious natural resources for future generations.

## LONG POINT

Lat/Long: 48.2263, -122.6491
At end of Marine Dr, Coupeville

**Directions:** a) *From the north:* turn off Hwy 20, N onto Main St and E onto 9th St which becomes Parker Rd. Travel approximately 1.5 miles, turn L onto Portal Place and then L on Marine Dr, continuing 0.5 mile to the road end. *b) From the south:* turn off Hwy 20 onto Morris Rd, then L in 500 ft onto Parker Rd. Go 1 mile and turn R onto Portal Place and continue as above.

**Parking:** 8-10

**Adjoining public tideland:** 1.6 miles west to Captain Coupe Park, 0.9 mile east.

This beautiful stretch of flat beach boasts magnificent views of Mount Baker and Oak Harbor. Great blue herons and eagles can be seen feeding at low tide. The point tends to collect driftlogs and reaching the beach may require climbing over them.

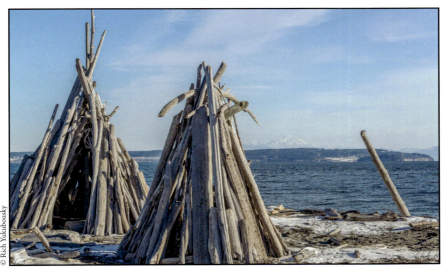

Long Point

### We're choking on plastic

We're plasticizing our globe and destroying life because items designed for single and short-term use are being made from a material that never goes away. Our oceans are awash in plastic, composing three-quarters of beach litter worldwide. The problem surrounds us. For

*(continued)*

example, in Puget Sound, 12 samples of beach sand revealed an average of 1,776 pieces of invisible microplastics per 3-foot-square sampling plot. The highest concentration of plastics by number was in Everett (UW News, June 2017).

Plastic is manufactured of molecules not found in nature. It doesn't biodegrade and when exposed to air, water, and wave action, it breaks into smaller and smaller pieces, eventually invisible but still deadly. At sea, it settles randomly in plankton blooms, sea grasses, and seaweeds. On shore, it nestles into sand, lodges in vegetation, and accumulates under driftwood.

Plastic has become part of the global food chain. Tiny amounts are eaten by phytoplankton and zooplankton, which in turn are eaten by marine animals and sea birds. Filter-feeding shellfish consume it. Humans also consume it. BPA, a plastic component in some water bottles, has been found in the urine of 95% of American adults tested and in 90% of the cord blood of newborn infants. Microscopic fibers too fine to filter out are found in salt, sugar, honey, beer, and both tap and bottled water. Even large plastic items, such as garbage bags and soda bottles, are scooped up by gray whales as they hunt ghost shrimp along coastal shores.

Recycling often isn't a viable solution, but you can help. Stopping the use of plastic will reduce plastic production; try to purchase and use less.

1. The most common items in ocean trash are single-use food related plastic, so whenever possible, carry your own reusable containers and utensils and avoid plastic straws.
2. Find products made of alternative materials, such as reusable glass storage containers and stainless water bottles.
3. Synthetic fabrics shed millions of microfibers into each wash load, so when you can, choose clothing made from natural fibers.
4. Do the best you can to avoid buying over-packaged products and deliver foam peanuts and bubble wrap (neither is recyclable) back to shipping stores.
5. Dispose of plastic products judiciously, discarding them in appropriate places, not onto waterways, beaches, trails, and roadways.
6. Help clean up. Whenever you're going to a beach, take a bag to carry out plastics you pick up. Join an organization to help out. On Whidbey and Camano Islands, programs like Washington State University Extension's "On the Beach" are open to all volunteers for group beach cleanups.

Essentially, reduce + reuse + rethink. Educate yourself and others.

**Directions:** *a) From the north:* From Hwy 20 before reaching the traffic light at Coupeville, turn R onto Ebey Rd (just before the electrical substation). In 0.25 mile continue straight on Ebey Rd past Terry Rd. In another 1.2 miles, at the bottom of a short hill, the parking area is on the R. *b) From the south:* Turn L at Coupeville traffic light onto S Main St. In 0.25 mile at stop sign turn R onto Terry Rd. In 0.25 mile turn L onto Ebey Rd, continue 1.2 miles to parking area on R. (Directions to walking access from Cemetery Rd are below.)

**Parking:** 10+ A Discover Pass is required to park in designated lot. A few roadside spaces are available as well. 

**Adjoining public tideland:** Northwest 4 miles to Fort Ebey beach access and southeast 3.5 miles to Fort Casey State Park/Keystone Harbor.

Ebey's Landing is part of Ebey's Landing National Historical Reserve and provides excellent exploration of bluffs and beaches. From the parking area (the Landing), walkable beaches stretch far to the northwest. Before leaving on a long beach hike, check your tide tables. Tides in the Pacific Northwest are described as being semidiurnal mixed tides; two high tides and two low tides of mixed heights in a 24-hour time period. An extremely high tide, coupled with wind-driven waters, can create a very hazardous situation that leaves the beachcomber stranded with no upland access.

A trail ascends stairs and climbs the bluff, curving along the top with commanding views of the beach below, Admiralty Inlet, the Olympic Mountains, and both Mount Rainier and Mount Baker. The plant community on this bluff is one of the few remaining examples of a natural, coastal prairie ecosystem. Few comparable areas remain in our state, most having been lost in the last 150 years to farming and bluff-top homes. The trail follows the bluff about 1¾ miles before descending via switchbacks to the beach at the west end of Perego's Lagoon, a brackish, saltwater wetland located between beach and bluff. The round trip is about 3½ miles. Note that in some areas the trail contains loose sand and steep slopes and care should be taken on your descent. Dogs must be leashed on all trails.

Ebey's Landing can also be reached on foot from Cemetery Rd. Turn W off Hwy 20 onto Sherman Rd and continue straight on Cemetery Rd. Park on the L at the Prairie Overlook opposite the far end of the cemetery; or continue between hedges to additional parking and Ebey's Reserve Trail Portal kiosk. Ebey's Prairie Ridge Trail starts past the vault toilet and follows the edge of fields for 0.8 mile to reach Ebey's Bluff. The trail passes the historic

Jacob & Sarah Ebey House and the Ebey Blockhouse, which are open to the public during the summer months; check with Ebey's Landing National Historical Reserve for details. The historic Sunnyside Cemetery is also interesting to explore.

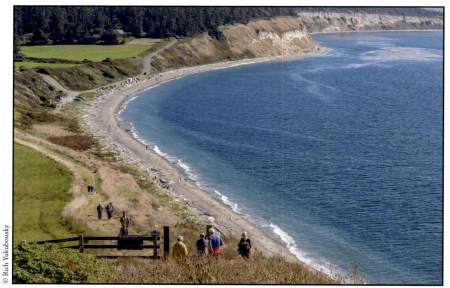

© Rich Yukubousky

*Ebey's Landing*

## Ebey's Landing National Historical Reserve

The tug of history is everywhere on central Whidbey Island. The picturesque seaside village of Coupeville, with its false-front buildings and historic wharf, sits only a short distance from rich natural prairies and woodlands dotted with turn-of-the-century homes and working farms, sweeping vistas of mountains and sea, old frontier blockhouses, and a marvelous pioneer cemetery. Equally important is what isn't there: urban sprawl and built-up development.

Central Whidbey's natural beauty and historic roots have been preserved for future generations by a unique experiment: the 17,400-acre Ebey's Landing National Historical Reserve. This first-of-its-kind national park is built on the concept of maintaining mostly private ownership and use of the land while employing tax incentives and other strategies to preserve its character.

# FORT CASEY HISTORICAL STATE PARK
Lat/Long: 48.1583, -122.6813
1280 Engle Rd, Coupeville

**Directions:** Located next to Keystone Harbor. *a) From the north:* From Hwy 20 at Coupeville traffic light, turn S onto Main St, which becomes Engle Rd. Travel 3.5 miles to park entrance on S side, after Camp Casey and before the Coupeville Ferry terminal. *b) From the south:* Go 5 miles N of Greenbank on Hwy 525 to the intersection with Race Rd. Turn W onto Hwy 20 (Wanamaker Rd) toward the Coupeville Ferry landing. After 1.75 miles, the highway makes a 90° turn S, then turns 90° W to parallel the south shore of Crockett Lake. The park entrance is on the L, 0.25 mile past the ferry terminal.

**Parking:** Parking is plentiful. A Discover Pass is required.

Of all the ships to sail past Whidbey Island's Admiralty Head into Puget Sound in the last three centuries, none left a greater legacy than *HMS Discovery* in 1792, under the command of Captain George Vancouver. Vancouver named the high bluff Admiralty Head. The commanding site soon had a lighthouse and then a coastal artillery post, Fort Casey, which still enthralls visitors with its historic guns and spectacular view over Admiralty Inlet.

Two miles of shoreline beach are available for walking, and a wide parade field atop the windblown bluff is popular for kite flying. The park has 1.8 miles of hiking trails. Admiralty Head Lighthouse, built in 1901 to replace the original wooden structure, is a historic landmark and interpretive center, open seasonally. A trail behind the lighthouse leads through a compost demonstration site. A boat launch is available at Fort Casey State Park (see Site 30), but it requires additional permitting to use in addition to the Discover Pass needed to park.

## Ebey's Prairie agriculture

Hiking trails, overlooks, county roads, and numerous public access points give visitors captivating views of the rich farm fields of Ebey's Prairie on central Whidbey. Today, some farmers of central Whidbey still work land claims that date back in their families to the mid-1800s.

Three large natural prairies, once lake beds, were left behind when glacial ice receded. Now agricultural land, farmers plant diversified crops such as grasses and alfalfa for livestock forage, grains, small acreages of vegetables, and a variety of grass and vegetable seed crops.

<table>
<tr><td>

**Site 30**

</td><td>

## KEYSTONE JETTY (Fort Casey State Park)
Lat/Long: 48.1583, -122.6716
1400 Hwy 20, Coupeville

</td></tr>
</table>

**Directions:** Located alongside the Coupeville Ferry landing, S of Coupeville. Follow directions to Site 29. The parking area and boat launch are on the E shore of the ferry harbor.

**Parking:** 50+ A Discover Pass is required to park here. An additional permit is needed to use the boat launch. 🍴 🚻 🪑 🛶 ➤ 🏕

**Adjoining public tideland:** Jetty and Park only.

The constructed Keystone Jetty has interrupted the natural longshore movement of sediment. This structure causes beach accretion (addition) on the up-drift side (ferry channel) and beach erosion on the down-drift side.

The jetty, part of the protected Keystone Conservation Area, is a popular dive site and displays a vast collection of lingcod, rockfish, sea anemones, and an array of other invertebrates among the rocks. If you plan to use this site for your next dive, it's advised that you familiarize yourself with the hazards of this location and always check daily weather and tidal conditions. Use caution, especially when venturing out on the jetty during wet weather or heavy wave action.

The substrate at this beach could be difficult for some beachgoers to navigate, with cobble closer to the water and larger rocks and driftwood higher up.

Enjoy views of the Olympic Mountains and the ship traffic in Admiralty Inlet.

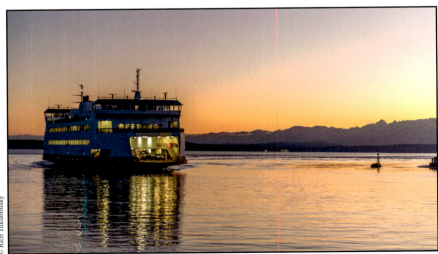

© Rich Yukubousky

*Ferry entering Keystone Harbor to Coupeville ferry dock*

## Fort Casey Underwater State Park—a hidden treasure

A wonderland of marine plants and animals, brilliantly colorful and fabulously diverse, is just out of sight in the dark waters next to the 250-foot Keystone Jetty at Fort Casey. Scuba divers from across Washington, British Columbia, and the Northwest travel here to find and photograph 50-year-old rockfish, mature ling cod as big as children, giant Pacific octopus, wolf eels, buffalo sculpin, kelp greenling, great cabezon, and surf perch. Adding to the rich display are large plumose anemones, bull kelp, and eelgrass, as well as countless varieties of sea cucumbers, crabs, sea stars, barnacles, and tube worms. The anemone garden covers thousands of square feet. The cold waters and swift currents around Keystone Jetty ensure a rich food supply for these plants and animals that find shelter in a habitat ranging from sand and cobble to large boulders.

In the early 1970s, Washington State Parks & Recreation Commission established Fort Casey Underwater State Park as part of a system of underwater parks to provide high-quality dive sites for recreation and to preserve Washington's marine resources. Keystone Conservation Area is a Marine Protected Area of the Washington Department of Fish & Wildlife. It lies entirely inside the boundaries of the underwater park and is closed to all consumptive recreational activities.

Because of the powerful currents, nearby fishing and boating activity, ferry crossing, and other hazards, divers are strongly advised to ask for a thorough safety briefing about this area before setting out. Experienced divers who know this site may be located by inquiring at local dive shops.

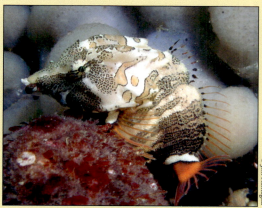

*Grunt sculpin at Keystone*

**KEYSTONE SPIT** (Fort Casey State Park)
Lat/Long: west entrance 48.1620, -122.6577
east entrance 48.1635, -122.6471
1400 Hwy 20, Coupeville

**Directions:** Follow directions for Site 29 and continue E of the ferry dock past the private residences. At two points along the spit, vehicles may enter parking areas via gravel roads, one located 0.6 mile E of the ferry slip and the other 1.1 miles E of the ferry slip, a short way E of milepost 14. From the south, the easternmost Keystone Spit parking entry is 0.5 mile W of Site 32.

**Parking:** 50+ A Discover Pass is required to park here.

**Adjoining public tideland:** 1.5 miles. Bordered by the homes just east of the Jetty and by Keystone Rd.

Keystone Spit, part of Fort Casey State Park, is a 2-mile stretch of land separating Admiralty Inlet and Crockett Lake. Along the tidelands is an enormous amount of driftwood blown up onto the backshore by prevailing winds. Crockett Lake is a 700-acre mixture of salt and fresh water marshes, mudflats, open water, and grasslands providing rich feeding for a variety of birdlife. It's designated as an Important Bird Area for Washington state because large numbers of shorebirds use it as a stopover during their southbound (early July-October) migrations. Twenty species of ducks and 34 species of shorebirds have been recorded here. These birds draw raptors such as peregrine falcons, merlins, short-eared owls, northern harriers, and bald eagles. Great blue herons forage here during breeding season. A platform for bird watching is south of milepost 14 at the west end of the eastern vehicle access. Explore the spit on foot by walking the central road and pathways.

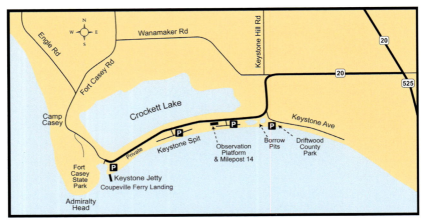

*Keystone Spit pullouts and observation platform*

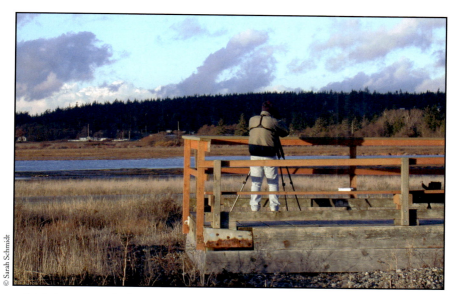

*Bird observation platform at Keystone Spit*

## Seven Island County sites listed as essential for birds

The Important Bird Areas (IBA) program is a worldwide effort to identify key places of importance for maintaining healthy bird populations. In Washington State, 75 areas have been designated as IBAs. These critical landscapes, considered "sites most essential for long-term conservation of birds," were chosen using standard biological criteria and review by expert ornithologists. The list includes seven Important Bird Areas in Island County: Deception Pass Marine Foraging Area, Crescent Harbor Marshes, Penn Cove, Crockett Lake, Deer Lagoon, Port Susan Bay, and Skagit Bay.

In addition, the Greater Skagit/Stillaguamish Delta system (91,000 acres of Port Susan and Skagit Bays) is recognized as a Western Hemisphere Shorebird Reserve Network (WHSRN) site of Regional importance. It's used annually during winter periods and also during spring and fall migration by over 60,000 shorebirds.

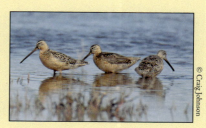

*Dowitchers*

**Directions:** *a) From the south:* Go 5 miles N of Greenbank on Hwy 525 to the intersection with Race Rd. Turn W onto Hwy 20 (Wanamaker Rd) toward the Coupeville Ferry landing. After 1.75 miles, the road makes a 90° turn S. In another 0.25 mile, where Keystone Rd turns 90° between the spit and Crockett Lake, go straight ahead into park at road end. *b) From the north:* Follow directions for Site 29. Continue E past ferry 2 miles. When highway turns 90° L, instead turn R into the park.

**Parking:** 20 ⬛ 🛬 🚶 🛶 🐦 ⛺ Toilet is seasonal.

**Adjoining public tideland:** In front of park and 1½ miles west along Keystone Spit.

The shore of this aptly-named ¾-acre park at the east end of Keystone Spit is piled thickly with driftwood, a reminder that this area is also a catch-point for drifting marine debris. In season it's a popular fishing site. Ducks are often seen in the two gravel borrow pits west of the parking lot; look north towards the Crockett Lake Wetlands Preserve for more bird viewing. The park offers a view of the snowy peaks of the Olympic mountains and the busy shipping lanes between Whidbey Island and Fort Flagler. At lower tides, 1½ miles of beach walking is available along Keystone Spit to the west.

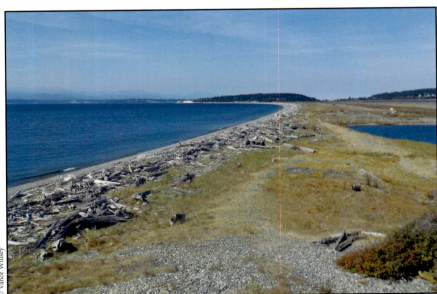

© Vance Willsey

*Driftwood Beach Park*

# LWD–you can't miss it

That tangle of sun-bleached logs pushed far onto the backshore by extreme tides and storms is what scientists call LWD: large woody debris. While it may look like a mess, it's actually a sophisticated shock absorber and much more.

Most of those logs started out as trees along riverbanks or bluffs. These trees eventually became undercut and fell into the water. They floated to their present location and became knit together in a complex web that absorbs wave energy and helps hold soils, thereby reducing erosion of the shore. On the backshore, they both trap and release organic material, moisture, and nutrients to help sustain plant life. These logs also provide spots for both resting and roosting for a variety of birds and other wildlife and also places for aquatic invertebrates to attach themselves.

Tempting as it may be to take home some driftwood from the beach, laws prohibit its removal in many jurisdictions – and it makes sense to leave it in place. Woody debris in general helps stabilize shorelines, and even small pieces provide useful shelter and habitat for beach-dwelling creatures.

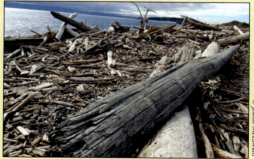

*Driftwood Park LWD*

| Site 33 | **LEDGEWOOD BEACH ACCESS** (Driftwood Way) |
|---|---|
| | Lat/Long: 48.1429, -122.6045 |
| | 1846 Driftwood Way, Coupeville |

**Directions**: Turn W off Hwy 525 onto Ledgewood Beach Rd. At T intersection, turn N onto Fircrest Ave for 0.5 mile, then W onto Seaward Way. Wind downhill to make sharp hairpin turn R onto Driftwood Way and follow it N 600 feet to parking area on L. Beach is accessed by a steep ramp.

**Parking**: 5-6 ⬤ ⬤ ⬤ ⬤

**Adjoining public tideland:** North 1 mile, south 1.5 miles.

Beach and coastline stability depend on the capability of coastal features to resist changes by geological, environmental, or human-made events. Ledgewood Beach shows evidence of stability failure in all three. Excessive rains followed by a cold freeze caused the uplands to slough and slide in December of 1990, damaging two homes north of the parking lot; another slide occurred there in January 1997. More recently, a March 2013 Ledgewood-Bonair landslide occurred 200 yards south of the beach access. The beach, bluffs, and bulkheads that have fallen into the surf show evidence of continued erosion and recession from shoreline wave action. This beach can be very dangerous 0.25 mile north of the beach access due to serious calving (large chunks of land falling) off the bluff. When in this area, it's safest to always walk near the water's edge. There's no beach at high tide.

## Birds of the bluffs

The shores of Island County include miles of steep, erosional bluffs. In sections bare of vegetation you may have noticed round or oval holes; these are the nesting burrows of belted kingfishers, rough-winged swallows, and pigeon guillemots.

### Kingfishers hover and dive

While walking the beach, you may hear the reverberating rattle-like call of a belted kingfisher. This bird can be observed hovering high above the water (an osprey does this also) looking for prey. The belted kingfisher is blue and white, with a white ring around its neck, a slate blue breast band, and a shaggy crest on the back of its head. The female sports an additional rust-red belly band, a rare case among birds where the female of the species is more colorful than the male. If you see a kingfisher flying overhead, watch its wings beat a Morse-code pattern with flashing white wing patches.

Stocky and short-legged, this bird's power is in its large head and sharp bill. The king of fishers hovers over water and then dives headfirst to catch prey in its bill. Emerging from the water, the bird flies back to a perch. There it juggles the meal—usually a fish or aquatic invertebrate—into position and gulps it down.

In spring, belted kingfishers dig nesting burrows in sandy bluffs. They use their front claws, with two forward-pointing toes fused together for added strength, and their strong bills to dig out holes. The burrows typically reach three to six feet into the bank, but some nesting holes extend up to 15 feet.

*(continued)*

## Birds of the bluffs continued

### Swallows hunt in the air

The northern rough-winged swallow is an aerial artist Its diet is 100% insects, which it usually catches in flight but occasionally plucks from the ground. Pale brown above and white below with a dingy brown breast, these 5½-inch birds nest in a burrow or cavity. They use deserted kingfisher burrows, rodent holes, and ready-made niches in bridges, wharves, culverts, and other structures.

### Pigeon guillemots swim in groups

In spring and summer, you may spot groups of velvety-black seabirds with white wing patches and bright red feet swimming near shore and emitting high-pitched, piping whistles and trilled songs. This is the pigeon guillemot, the only species in the alcid family (which includes puffins, murres, and auklets) that breeds on Whidbey and Camano Islands. They lay their two eggs in burrows, which often are abandoned kingfisher burrows. Look for their holes in sandy bluffs, often among the roots of bluff-top vegetation. Watch for their synchronized courtship flights as pairs rocket over the water, turning as one. In July and August, the parents carry single fish to their one or two chicks in the burrow.

Volunteers from Whidbey Audubon Society, working with the Island County Marine Resources Committee, have been surveying about 1,000 pigeon guillemots in 27 colonies on Whidbey Island since 2004. Activities recorded include population counts, visiting burrows, and delivering food to burrows. The guillemots typically select bottom-dwelling fish like gunnels, pricklebacks, and sculpins to deliver to the young. Learn more and see videos at **pigeonguillemot.org**.

Watch for these fascinating birds the next time you walk the beach under our bluffs. To help this species maintain a viable population, detour around the birds if they are resting on the beach, walk quickly past their colonies, and keep your dog on a leash. Because pigeon guillemots breed throughout Puget Sound, this species has been selected as an indicator species by the Puget Sound Partnership.

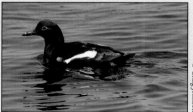

*Pigeon guillemot*

**HIDDEN BEACH** (Crane's Landing Drive)
Lat/Long: 48.1288, -122.5630
2269 Hidden Beach Dr, Greenbank

**Directions:** From Greenbank, turn E from Hwy 525 onto North Bluff Rd. In 2.25 miles turn R onto Neon Ln for a short block, then L on Crane's Landing Dr. Continue downhill around a long curve and veer L onto Hidden Beach Dr. The parking area is on L at bottom of the hill prior to reaching the end of the road. Past it is a private community club.

**Parking:** 12-14 🚗 🚶 🚤 ⛱

**Adjoining public tideland:** 730 feet to north only, along isolated cobble beach with overhanging trees. Private to south.

Hidden Beach is a beautiful, small stretch of cobble and gravel beach, lined with several old pilings and large rocks. There is a small, unpaved boat access that would be appropriate for hand-carried boats. Posted information reveals a restoration project in the works at this beach to remove the rocks and pilings and result in improved habitat for local fish and birds.

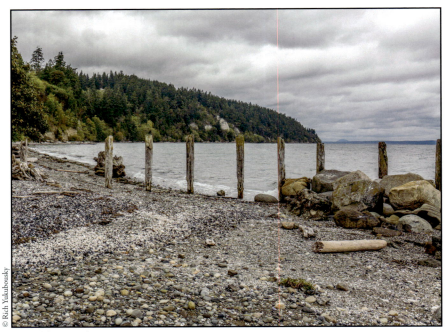

© Rich Yukubousky

*Hidden Beach*

### WONN ROAD
Lat/Long: 48.1046, -122.5716
End of Wonn Rd. Park at Greenbank Farm,
765 Wonn Road, Greenbank

**Directions:** From Hwy 525, turn E onto Wonn Road and in approximately 0.1 mile make your first L into Greenbank Farm. Park here and walk back out to Wonn Rd, then L towards North Bluff Rd. A beach access sign is seen where Wonn Rd meets North Bluff Rd. Continue to the road end.

**Parking:** 0 on site. Parking is at Greenbank Farm, approximately a two-block walk. Please do not park on residential streets.

**Adjoining public tideland:** Approximately 25 feet.

This is a sheltered access point for non-motorized watercraft to the west side of the mouth of Holmes Harbor. Loading and unloading non-motorized watercraft is allowed but parking is not. Public access is literally a half-width road end since an agreement was reached between the county and property owners. Signage is substantial and cautions users about very tight boundaries on either side of the narrow public access.

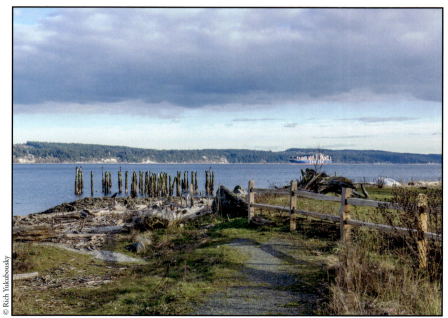

© Rich Yukubousky

*Wonn Road beach access is 25 feet wide where the trail meets the beach; there is no public tideland either side.*

## Septic systems impact oysters, clams, mussels

As in rural areas everywhere, most sewage in Island County is treated on site in household septic systems and drainfields. When these systems are overwhelmed or poorly maintained, bacteria can make their way into marine waters and contaminate shellfish beds and beaches.

Shellfish are filter feeders that subsist by consuming tiny particles in the water, so contamination makes shellfish unsafe to eat. Every year, beaches are closed or restricted due to fecal contamination from failed septic systems.

Homeowners, renters, and visitors can help by following some preventive practices: 1) Minimize household water use to avoid taxing the system; 2) keep grease, cigarettes, chemicals, and other microbe-killing materials out of septic systems; 3) limit use of the garbage disposal; 4) use drain screens on all sinks; 5) keep kitty litter and pet waste out of the system; and 6) routinely maintain the septic system by inspecting it every one to three years, depending on the type of system on the property.

Contact the Island County Health Department for more specific information.

**Site 36A**

## LAGOON POINT NORTH (Westcliff Drive)
Lat/Long: 48.0826, -122.6105
95 Westcliff Drive, Greenbank

**Directions:** *a) From the north:* Turn W off Hwy 525 onto Smugglers Cove Rd (0.7 mile N of Greenbank). In 2.7 miles, turn R onto Westcliff Dr. At bottom of hill drive straight toward shore into gravel parking area. Signs mark private property to either side of the beach. *b) From the south:* Just N of Freeland, turn off Hwy 525 W onto Bush Point Rd, which becomes Smugglers Cove Rd. In 6.6 miles turn L onto Westcliff Dr and follow directions above.

**Parking:** 8-10 ⬛ ✈ ⬛ 🅿 Toilet is seasonal.

**Adjoining public tideland:** 397 feet.

This is a very popular salmon fishing beach. Lagoon Point offers views of the Olympic mountains, Port Townsend, and a very active shipping lane. A portable toilet is available during fishing season only (August 1 to November 30). To ensure you stay within the public access, please consult the signage displayed by Island County Parks department.

**LAGOON POINT SOUTH** (Salmon Street)
Lat/Long: 48.0718, -122.6132
Next to 60 Salmon Street, Greenbank

**Directions:** Follow Site 36A directions, turning off Smugglers Cove Rd onto Westcliff Dr. Turn L onto Lagoon View Dr, then R onto Salmon St. At end of Salmon St continue straight across intersection into access.

**Parking:** 2-3

**Adjoining public tideland:** 30 feet only. Please respect privately owned beach to either side.

This limited beach access is one of the better salmon and steelhead fishing sites in Island County. If you're not into fishing but are into waves, this beach is a great place to observe and ponder while enjoying a panoramic view of the Olympic mountain range.

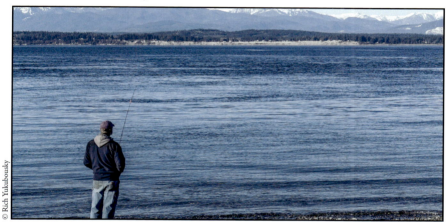

*Lagoon Point South*

## Whidbey Island's west side—paradise for shore fishers

One look at the map tells the story: Whidbey Island sits at the entrance to Puget Sound, so nearly every salmon, steelhead, and sea-run cutthroat trout migrating from Puget Sound rivers to the ocean and back will swim past Whidbey shores. Many of the returning southbound fish hug the shore to feast on the teeming forage fish that lay their eggs on Whidbey's nearshore eelgrass and healthy beaches. As a result, many anglers consider Whidbey Island's west side to be the state's best bet for shore fishing.

*(continued)*

## Whidbey Island's west side—paradise continued

Anglers enjoy year-round opportunities to fish miles of uncrowded public shoreline in the island's many parks and other public access areas. They look for aquatic vegetation and rocky or gravelly shoreline and cast lures or bait with traditional salmon rods, fly gear, or spinning reels. Fly fishers typically are seeking the feisty sea-run cutthroat trout, which range from 13 to 20 inches and come as close to shore as a few feet of the water's edge. Cutthroat migrate back to Puget Sound's larger rivers in the fall, and when caught in saltwater, must be released alive.

For silver salmon, pink salmon (also called humpies), and winter steelhead, shore anglers favor traditional spinning or salmon gear. Flies may be used but most anglers use bait such as plug-cut herring or Buzz Bombs, weighted jigs, or a local favorite called the Bush Point rig. Salmon and steelhead typically are found in 4 to 6 feet of water, so anglers cast out about 40 feet. Pinks run in odd-numbered years. Wild Chinook, wild coho, and wild steelhead are protected species, and must be released alive.

Before planning any fishing trip, anglers should make sure they are properly licensed. Fishing regulations vary seasonally and can change frequently, so in addition, carefully consult the official Washington Sport Fishing Rules, published by the WDFW, available at many hardware stores and other outlets where fishing tackle is sold. This publication provides detailed information on seasons, limits, and other rules. The booklet is also available online, with updates and notices, and there is a FishWA app.

## Site 37 — SOUTH WHIDBEY STATE PARK

Lat/Long: 48.0571, -122.5954
4128 Smugglers Cove Road, Freeland

**Directions:** *a) From the north:* Turn R off Hwy 525 onto Smugglers Cove Rd. Proceed 4 miles to park entrance on R side of Smugglers Cove Rd. *b) From the south:* Just N of Freeland turn L onto Bush Point Rd, which becomes Smugglers Cove Rd. The park entrance is on L in 5 miles.

**Parking:** About 50 spaces. A Discover Pass is required to park here.

**Adjoining public tideland:** 600 feet. Although the park has 600 feet of public tidelands, at the time of publication, the Beach Trail is closed indefinitely due to bluff erosion. The beach can be reached by foot from Site 38 or by boat.

South Whidbey is a 380-acre, day-use park offering views of Admiralty Inlet and the Olympic Mountains and 3.5 miles of hiking trails, including through the Classic U Forest, one of the best stands of old-growth forest remaining in Island County. This forest trail is east of Smugglers Cove Rd. Walk among giant Douglas fir, Sitka spruce, western hemlock and western red cedar trees, including a 500-year-old cedar.

Throughout spring and summer, blooming wildflowers and shrubs add color to the park and produce salmonberries, huckleberries, and black cap raspberries.

Campsites have been closed at this site due to tree fall risk, a natural side effect of the life cycle of old-growth forests. The former campground roads offer ADA accessible trails through forest rich with birdlife.

## Forage fish "fuel" the marine food web

Three tiny fish known as forage fish—surf smelt, sand lance, and herring—cruise the waters of Camano and Whidbey islands in vast numbers. These three are Puget Sound's pre-eminent forage fish, a vital link in the marine food chain because they lay a banquet for salmon, seabirds, and marine mammals. This provides a transfer of energy between primary and secondary producers, such as plankton, to top predators, such as seabirds and larger fish. For centuries, forage fish have been an important subsistence food for tribal cultures and continue to be harvested both recreationally and commercially. Herring are a favorite bait for recreational salmon fishing. Beach walkers sometimes observe shifting clouds of these little fish darting in the shallows just beyond the water's edge or spot them below over-water piers.

Pacific sand lance and surf smelt lay their eggs near the high tide line on the protected sandy gravel beaches of Camano and Whidbey Islands at certain times of the year. Pacific herring spawn directly on the lush vegetation in the many intertidal eelgrass beds. These same eelgrass beds offer refuge and shelter to juvenile salmon.

Sand lance and surf smelt benefit from beaches with low wave energy and overhanging trees to shade their eggs from overheating in the midday sun. They also benefit from beaches relatively free of human-made structures that can concentrate wave energy, which scours away spawning gravels. All forage fish and juvenile salmon benefit from healthy eelgrass beds.

*(continued)*

## Forage fish continued

Forage fish are so important to salmon and other marine life that Island County Marine Resources Committee took a step toward preserving healthy habitats by mapping every beach on Camano and Whidbey Islands where forage fish are known to spawn. The map can be found online under the search title "Island County: Marine Shellfish and Forage Fish." Greater understanding of these fish and the habitat they require is aiding efforts to restore salmon populations.

**Site 38**

## BUSH POINT BOAT LAUNCH
Lat/Long: 48.0335, -122.6032
231 East Spyglass Drive, Freeland

**Directions:** From Hwy 525 just N of Freeland, turn W onto Bush Point Rd (becomes Smugglers Cove Rd) for 2.7 miles, fork L onto Scurlock Rd for 0.75 mile, then L onto Spyglass Dr. Public access and boat launch are on R at bottom of hill. Continue L around the corner to large paved parking lot.

**Parking:** 12 spaces are available: 10 vehicles with trailers, 2 ADA accessible.

**Adjoining public tideland:** 15 feet either side of boat launch; public beach begins 400 feet N.

The boat ramp provides the best deep-water access on the west side of south Whidbey. This site is managed by the Port of South Whidbey. A minimum tide of 0.0' is recommended for boat launching at this site, and note that weather and currents can be severe, so check ahead and plan accordingly.

The public access includes about 15 feet either side of boat launch. No stopping is allowed on the beach in front of the private houses on either side of the access, but you can walk 400 feet N along the tideline past the houses to reach a long public beach at the foot of the bluff, popular for fishing or beach walking. There is an expansive view west along Admiralty Inlet between the Olympic Peninsula and Whidbey Island. This is a great location to look for whales from shore.

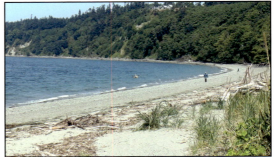

*Bush Point Boat Launch beach area*

# Orcas–our intelligent, sensitive marine neighbors

Few creatures inspire more outright awe than orcas, sometimes called killer whales (they, like dolphins, are members of the toothed whale family, Delphinidae). These magnificent mammals are gifted with high intelligence, complex communication, close family structure, and lifespans of 50 years or more. They live, eat, relax, and travel in groups, having much in common with their dominant terrestrial neighbor–humankind. Puget Sound's orcas live in family units called pods led by the eldest female.

The Pacific Northwest is home to two ecotypes of orcas. Biggs (transient) orcas generally live in smaller pods or matrilines and exclusively eat marine mammals; conversely, Resident orcas live in larger extended families and exclusively eat fish. The two groups are genetically distinct and don't socialize, mate, or communicate with one another.

In the waters of Whidbey and Camano Islands, most orcas sighted from late fall through mid-winter belong to the three pods of the Southern Resident population: J, K, and L pods. This group communicates with calls completely different from the calls of other groups, even those found in the same waters, and probably has lived in Puget Sound since the glaciers retreated more than 10,000 years ago. The population has ranged in recent decades from about 80 to 100. In 2005, with fewer than 90 individuals remaining, the Southern Residents were federally listed as endangered.

Unlike some other orca populations, the Southern Residents rely heavily on Chinook salmon for their diet. Declining salmon populations and increasing pollution are believed to be major contributors to the stress on the Southern Residents. As of July 1, 2019, this population has dropped to 73. These orcas who historically frequented the San Juan islands and BC gulf islands almost daily in summer months, now only occasionally visit the core waters of their designated Critical Habitat: Puget Sound, Georgia Strait, and the inland reach of the Strait of Juan de Fuca. This change is likely due to the continued decline in Chinook salmon. As populations shift, more mammal-eating transients are feeding in Puget Sound, and the resident salmon-eating orcas are spending more time along the outer coast.

Humpback and minke whales are also seen in these waters.

## Site 39

**BUSH POINT** (Sandpiper Rd)
Lat/Long: 48.0323, -122.6054
End of Sandpiper Rd, Freeland

**Directions:** Follow Site 38 directions onto Spyglass Dr. At bottom of hill follow road to L, and at T intersection, turn R onto Sandpiper Rd to road end.

**Parking:** 2-4 Parking is very limited; please do not park in front of houses or block access to driveways. ⛵ 🐟

**Adjoining public tideland:** 45 feet, in front of road end only.

Don't access areas to south and north as these are privately owned beaches and tidelands. The beach and tidelands fronting on the lighthouse are also privately owned by homeowners and not available for access. This limited-access site has been used for years as a salmon fishing beach.

---

### Report stranded marine mammals

Seals, sea lions, whales, dolphins, and porpoises sometimes turn up dead or apparently stranded on Island County beaches. Seal pups should be left alone (see box pgs. 36-37). Report dead or stranded mammals in Island or Skagit Counties to the Central Puget Sound Marine Mammal Stranding Network: 1-866-ORCANET (866-672 2638).

Members of the network are volunteers authorized and trained by the National Marine Fisheries Service to investigate and collect scientific data that become part of a national database to track the health of our local marine population and environment, in addition to the effects of pollution within the food web. To join the network, call 1-866-ORCANET. (If you're reporting outside Island or Skagit County call the NOAA Fisheries hotline 1-866-767-6114.)

Should you spot a live whale or other marine mammal tangled in fishing gear, prompt reporting is the best way to assist it. In Washington, Oregon, and California, call the NOAA Fisheries entanglement reporting hotline at 1-877-SOS-WHALE (1-877-767-9425).

---

## Site 40

**MUTINY BAY VISTA** (Shore Meadows Rd)
Lat/Long: 48.0085, -122.5710
End of S Shore Meadows Rd, Freeland

**Directions:** Turn W off Hwy 525 onto Bush Point Rd. Travel 1.2 miles and turn S onto Shore Meadows Rd. Public access is at road end by the condominiums; parallel park on W side. A sidewalk leads SE downhill to beach access.

**Parking:** 7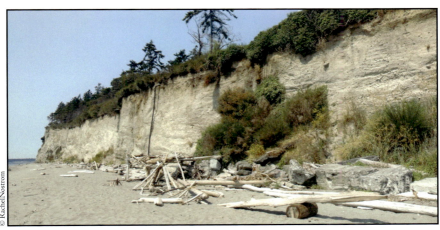

**Adjoining public tideland:** 295 feet, west from where the path reaches the beach to the tideland below the bluff in front of the parking area. The sidewalk and access were provided to the public as a condition of the condominium development. Please respect the privacy of those living in the condominiums.

This small beach is primarily sandy and provides great views of the Olympic mountains. It's a long distance to the water with a hand-carry boat. Marine birds can often be seen floating on Puget Sound looking for a meal, and pigeon guillemots nest in the nearby bluff. Please be mindful of noise levels and keep dogs on leash when birds are present.

*Mutiny Bay Vista*

## Site 41 — FREELAND PARK

Lat/Long: 48.0158, -122.5311
1535 East Shoreview Dr, Freeland

**Directions:** Located in Freeland at the head of Holmes Harbor. *a) From the north:* From Hwy 525 turn N onto Honeymoon Bay Rd then immediately E onto Shoreview Dr for 0.7 mile, uphill past Freeland Hall and down to park. Boat launch and park are marked with signs. *b) From the south:* Turn N at traffic light onto Main St, then L at stop sign onto E Harbor Rd. Fork L downhill on Stewart Dr, continue 0.3 mi. to park.

**Parking:** 30+

**Adjoining public tideland:** 720 feet of shoreline east of dock, 1,300 feet to west.

This 17-acre park, co-owned by Island County and the Port of South Whidbey and managed by Island County Parks, has a public moorage dock for day use. The tideflat slope is gradual; be cautious launching at mid to low tides to avoid being marooned in the mud.

When the tide is low, you can see patches of eelgrass growing in the soft sandy mud, a characteristic substrate at the heads of bays. Fish and many other organisms benefit by living in eelgrass habitat, including sponges, bryozoans, small worms, and tunicates. In Holmes Harbor, herring attach their eggs to the long eelgrass blades (see box pg. 29).

There is a small hiking trail as the park extends up the hill to the west with a picnic shelter; the trail passes Freeland Hall, built in 1907 and available for rental from Island County.

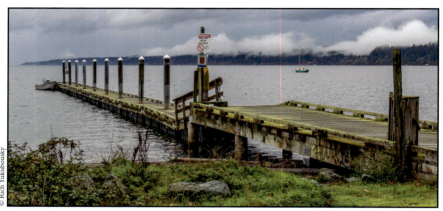

*Freeland Park dock*

## Site 42 — ROBINSON BEACH COUNTY PARK
### (Mutiny Bay Boat Launch)
Lat/Long: 47.9932, -122.5412
Robinson Rd end, Freeland

**Directions:** From Hwy 525 traffic light at Freeland turn S onto Fish Rd. Follow for 1 mile to T intersection and turn L onto Mutiny Bay Rd. After 0.3 mile, turn R onto Robinson Rd to beach access straight ahead. Please use the large parking area provided on the north side of Robinson Rd, 150 feet before beach.

**Parking:** 30+

**Adjoining public tideland:** Approximately 360 feet at boat ramp and in front of Robinson Beach.

This boat launch on a shallow, sandy bay is usable only for shallow-draft boats at optimal tides. The ramp frequently sands in, requiring a lot of maintenance. The launch at Bush Point is a better alternative for most watercraft, especially larger boats. Co-owned by Island County and the Port of South Whidbey, this access is managed by Island County Parks. Robinson Beach, parkland with 300 feet of waterfront located next to the boat launch, was gifted to the island by the Robinson family in 2013. Expected in summer 2020: accessible paved parking and trail to beach.

Because this shallow west-facing beach receives mid-day sun, its waters are sometimes surprisingly warm in summer, making it a popular sandy play area for children and families. It offers expansive views of ships passing through Admiralty Inlet and also the Olympic Mountains beyond.

This is a beautiful beach for an afternoon picnic on the sand, taking in the beauty of Puget Sound, or launching a kayak to explore Mutiny Bay.

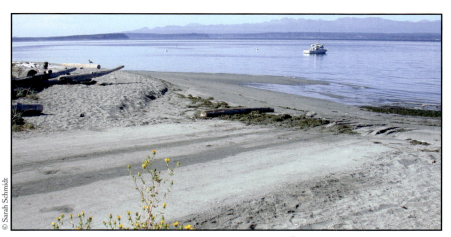

*Robinson Beach County Park*

| Site 43 | **MUTINY BAY SHORES** (Limpet Lane) |
|---|---|
| | Lat/Long: 47.9767, -122.5511 |
| | 1101 Limpet Lane, Freeland |

**Directions:** From Hwy 525 traffic light at Freeland, turn S onto Fish Rd. Follow for 1 mile to T intersection and turn L onto Mutiny Bay Rd. After 0.6 mile turn R onto Wahl Rd. At Ebb Tide Lane, turn R, then L onto Limpet Lane. From Mutiny Bay Rd to the access is 3 miles.

**Parking:** 1-2 Please park on the left side of Limpet Lane and take care to avoid blocking driveways. If the left side is full, overflow parking can be found along Ebb Tide Lane.

**Adjoining public tideland:** 950 feet to the NE.

Public access to this beach is the width of Limpet Lane from the road end to the mean high tide (MHT) line. Once you have reached the mean high tide line, public access is seaward from the MHT for 950 feet heading north. Please be mindful that all other parts of the beach are private and should not be disturbed, so keep dogs on leash and children close at hand. It's not unusual to see marine mammals at this beach; if so, keep a respectful distance and noise level.

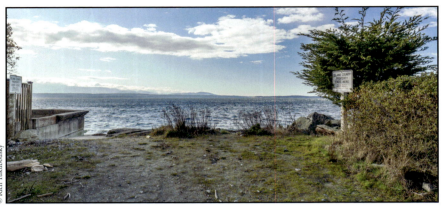

*Mutiny Bay Shores is a small public beach with close-up views of passing ships. The lower beach is mostly small, clean cobble transitioning to sand in the upper areas.*

## Site 44 — DOUBLE BLUFF BEACH
Lat/Long: 47.9816, -122.5143
End of Double Bluff Road, Freeland

**Directions:** Turn S off Hwy 525 (9 miles from Clinton) onto Double Bluff Rd. Follow 2 miles to parking lot at road end.

**Parking:** 24. Do not block driveway at access.

**Adjoining public tideland:** 2 miles to west, none to east.

This two-mile-long sandy beach is popular for family picnics and beach walking. An off-leash area for dogs begins beyond the windsock. Pay attention to off-leash guidelines and rules. Clean up after your dog (see box pg. 118). Signs point to an alternate entrance for dog owners; this may add an additional ¼ mile to your walk. A rinse station is provided near the parking lot. Pay attention to signs marking the beginning of the private beach and be respectful of residents.

At low tide, look for giant moon snails shoveling through the sand in search of clams to feast on. The collar-shaped egg cases are often mistaken for trash; however, they are left by the female moon snails to hatch, so leave them in place.

The sandy beach sediments come from the erosion of tall bluffs (see box next page) west of the access. Keep off the bluffs; eroding bluffs are not a safe place to play. Be aware that at higher tides there is no return to the public access when water reaches the foot of the bluff. High bluffs like these provide nesting burrows for pigeon guillemots, belted kingfishers, and rough-winged swallows (see box pgs. 70-71).

This beach is a wonderful place to explore the plethora of intertidal life at low tide and is excellent for year-round clamming, restricted to the cobble areas in the lower intertidal zone. Practice responsible clamming practices and beach etiquette (see pgs. 7-8 and 156-158).

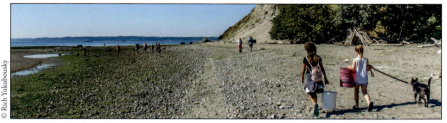

*Double Bluff Beach*

## Feeder bluffs provide spawning gravels

Glacially carved bluffs dominate large stretches of shoreline on Whidbey and Camano Islands. The erosion and redistribution of bluff material over time by wave and wind action are natural processes that help maintain healthy beaches and habitat for marine life. These bluffs continuously replenish beaches with sand and gravel that falls to the beach. It's distributed along the shoreline by littoral drift, the current that prevails on a specific segment of beach, determined by the angle at which waves routinely strike the shoreline at that point.

The gravel is the ideal size and consistency for use by forage fish to lay their eggs. Island County's abundant forage fish are a key part of the food chain that sustains salmon and other marine life.

The Island County Marine Resources Committee engaged geologists to identify and map all the feeder bluffs and drift cells on the county's 212 miles of shoreline. This 2005 study remains the most complete of its kind ever done and can be found along with successive studies at **islandcountymrc. org/projects** under "feeder bluff survey."

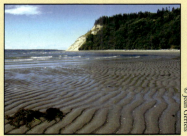

**Directions:** *a) From the south,* turn L off Hwy 525 onto Useless Bay Ave. In 0.4 mile, the road curves R onto Millman Rd. In 0.4 mile, turn L onto Deer Lagoon Rd; access is in 3 blocks at the road end; park on the side of this county road. *b) From the north,* turn R off Hwy 525 onto Double Bluff Rd. In 0.5 mile, turn L onto Millman Rd. In 0.7 mile turn R onto Deer Lagoon Rd, as above.

**Parking:** 8-10 on Deer Lagoon Rd. Don't block driveways and be considerate of neighbors. Please don't park on the side roads, Lori Dr and Gemini Dr, which are private.

Accessed from the south end of Deer Lagoon Rd, the lagoon consists of a landlocked area to the west and a tidal flat to the east, separated by a dike. A level footpath follows a watercourse through a wooded area, leading to the north end of the dike. Deer Lagoon offers views of superb wetland and estuary habitat with a great variety of birds that use the area for feeding and nesting, including waterfowl, shorebirds, songbirds, and, seasonally, a large flock of white pelicans. (To view the east half of the tidal area, go to Sunlight Beach, Site 46.) With much of Deer Lagoon adjacent to private land and the south end of the dike privately owned, please respect the neighbors. Dogs must be leashed and cleaned up after.

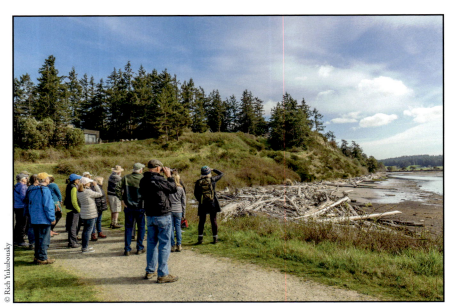

*Deer Lake Lagoon dike, looking east at tidal area*

# Sound Water Stewards' Intertidal Monitoring

Island County beaches are teeming with life and constantly changing with the ebb and flow of tides, winter storms, and human activity. Changes in intertidal life are key indicators of the health of upland areas as well as marine waters. Every year, volunteers from Sound Water Stewards diligently map the diversity of substrate, plants, and animals in the intertidal zone on Camano and Whidbey Island beaches. The sites range from quiet mudflats to wave-battered cobbles. It's challenging work, often on slippery terrain amid windy, rainy weather conditions, so beach profiling is a labor of love for these volunteers. They know they're building a priceless database to help marine scientists understand what stays the same and what changes on the beaches over time. The volunteers are adept at recognizing dozens of species of plants and creatures. This knowledge helps them rigorously adhere to a field-tested monitoring protocol based on accurate documentation.

Currently, Sound Water Stewards is the only group sequentially collecting and compiling such baseline information about Island County beaches. Members of Sound Water Stewards also join with partner organizations to do research in several areas of marine science. Projects have included observing pigeon guillemot colonies, tracking the invasive green crab, monitoring eelgrass and kelp beds, and sampling for the presence of toxic plankton.

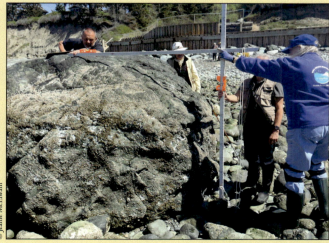

© Jeanie McElwain

## SUNLIGHT BEACH ACCESSES

Sunlight Beach Rd, Langley:
Two county-owned access points are suggested below.

**Directions:** From Hwy 525, turn S onto Bayview Rd. After a mile turn R onto Sunlight Beach Rd, driving slowly through this densely packed waterfront community.

**Access #1** (Lat/Long: 47.9908, -122.4821) is about 0.9 mile from Bayview Rd, between 2436 and 2440 Sunlight Beach Rd. This public access extends to both sides of the street, Useless Bay on the S side and to the lagoon on the N side.

**Parking:** 3 on the Useless Bay (S) side.

**Adjoining public tideland:** None on the lagoon side or to the east on bay side. On the Useless Bay side, public tidelands extend to the right of the beach access around to Deer Lagoon. Please respect neighbors and do not walk too close to beachfronts of homes.

**Access #2** (Lat/Long: 47.9916, -122.4846) Continue further along to county access just past 2402 Sunlight Beach Rd. A drive goes from the large paved area to the beach on the S side (see photo; park on the left side of the drive between the two houses with fences.)

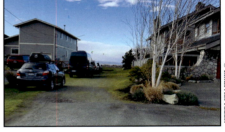
© Linda Ade Ridder

**Parking:** 5-6.

**Adjoining public tideland:** East to Access #1; west around to Deer Lagoon. Please respect neighbors and don't walk too close to beachfronts of homes. 🛶 🚶 🐦

Don't park on Sunlight Beach Road or in front of any homes.

The sandy beach on Useless Bay is reached from the S side of Sunlight Beach Rd. At higher tides, wind surfers, kayakers, and paddle boarders can launch from Access #2. Be cautioned that at low tide the water goes out a very long way and can come back in quickly. Know your tides before launching any watercraft so you don't become marooned. At low tides the bay becomes a vast expanse of sand flats stretching north to Double Bluff. No amenities are available at these sites. No beach fires.

This is a very popular birding area, both on the lagoon and bay sides of the road. Many species of birds use the lagoon and mudflats to dig for burrowing invertebrates. Deer Lagoon can be viewed from the N side of both public access points, but please don't park on this side. The mud of the shallow lagoon limits this side to view access only.

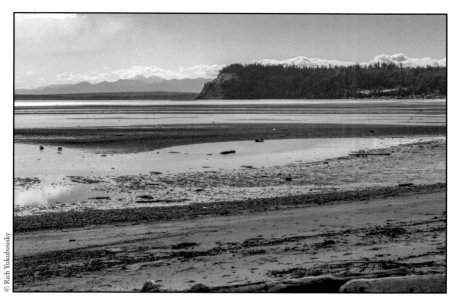

© Rich Yukubousky

*Sunlight Beach*

## Glacial erratics

Twenty thousand years ago, Whidbey and Camano Islands were covered by ice nearly a mile deep. This was the Puget Lobe of the Vashon Glacier, which flowed south from British Columbia. The direction in which the glacier flowed is reflected by the north-south orientation of most hills and valleys on Whidbey and Camano Islands, plainly visible on detailed elevation maps (see map pg. 134).

As the ice advanced, it carved large rocks from mountains and hills in the north and carried them south to where ice melted and randomly dropped this odd cargo. Many of these out-of-place glacial erratics, ranging from wheelbarrow-size to house-size, now sit in plain view on the fields and beaches of Whidbey and Camano Islands.

When located in the intertidal zone, these huge boulders provide a window into the diversity of sedentary marine life. The lower flanks of erratics house a mosaic of colorful, minute animal colonies known as bryozoans as well as pink coralline algae, calcareous tube worms, limpets, chitons, and giant barnacles. In the hollows under these boulders, you may find sea stars, colorful anemones, sea cucumbers, and other mobile sea creatures (see photo pg. 87).

## Site 47 — LONE LAKE COUNTY PARK (Fresh water)
### 5075 Lone Lake Rd, Langley

**Directions:** From Hwy 525, turn N at traffic light onto Bayview Rd. In 1.8 miles, turn W onto Andreason Rd. In 0.6 miles turn L on Lone Lake Rd. Follow Lone Lake Rd 0.3 miles until it ends at the parking area.

**Parking:** 20 plus 7 for boat trailers. 🔲 🔲 🔲 🔲

Lone Lake is popular for sailing, paddling, and fishing. There's a grassy area large enough to fly a kite or throw a frisbee. The lake has been beset by toxic algal blooms since summer 2017, and is now available for many activities only in cool seasons. Check warning signs and phone numbers. The anatoxin-a is particularly deadly and can cause death by respiratory paralysis; there is no rinse water for cleaning exposed pets. The access is owned by WDFW and managed by South Whidbey Parks and Recreation.

## Site 48 — GOSS LAKE COUNTY PARK (Fresh water)
### Lakeside Dr, Langley

**Directions:** From Hwy 525 in Freeland, turn N onto E Main St. In 0.2 miles, turn L onto E Harbor Rd. In 2.5 miles, turn R onto E Goss Lake Rd. In 1.7 miles, turn R on Traverse Rd. At stop sign, turn R on Lakeside Dr. Park is on L in 0.2 mile.

**Parking:** 8 🔲 🔲 🔲 🔲 🔲

This lake is popular with families, paddlers, distance swimmers, and fishermen. For fishing information, search online for "WDFW Fish Island Co Goss Lake." No petroleum-powered motors are allowed on Goss Lake. The access is owned by WDFW and managed by South Whidbey Parks and Recreation.

## Site 49 — LANGLEY SEAWALL PARK
### Lat/Long: at Anthes Ave 48.0413, -122.4090
### First St, Langley

**Directions:** Located in the City of Langley. Get to Langley from Hwy 525 by turning onto Bayview Rd, Maxwelton Rd, or Langley Rd. The waterfront park can be reached via Thomas Hladky Memorial Park at the intersection of First St and Anthes Ave or by stairs from the overlook on First St by the *Boy and His Dog* statue.

**Parking:** City streets offer ample parking, but there is no designated beach parking. 🔲 🔲 🔲 🔲 🔲

**Adjoining public tideland:** 1,000 feet.

Enjoy the view across Saratoga Passage to the bluffs at Camano Head with the *Boy and His Dog* statue located by the stairs on First Street. At low tide from this vantage point you can see sedimentary features made by currents and shifting sands. These include rill marks produced by water draining from the beach, swash marks composed of debris stranded by receding waves, and ripples produced by tidal currents. Migrating gray whales feed on ghost shrimp in the intertidal area during spring, leaving bathtub-sized depressions in the sand.

Seawall Park itself is a flat, grassy bank that runs above the shore between a concrete bulkhead and an embankment. Steps give access to the beach. While the sand close to the seawall is stable, it can get much softer the closer you get to the water, so walk with caution.

A public restroom is SE of the intersection of Second St and Anthes Ave.

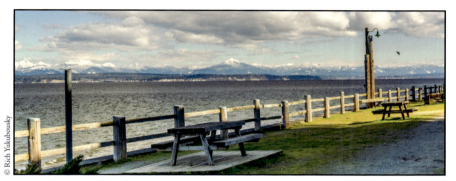

Langley Seawall Park

## Ghost shrimp–gray whales love 'em

If you've wondered what creates the little volcano-shaped mounds on beaches of mixed sand and mud substrate, the answer is ghost shrimp (*Neotrypaea californiensis*). Beneath the surface, these four-inch crustaceans carve out U-shaped tunnels where they feed on detritus in the mud. They are often joined in their burrows by other species, such as the small arrow goby fish, tiny pea crabs, scaleworms, and small clams. Humans may sink into the beaches where ghost shrimp reside because there are hundreds of tunnels

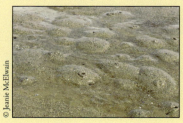

beneath their feet; these areas may be hundreds of feet wide. Solid ground may be two feet or more under the muddy sand. Therefore, volcano-shaped mounds and feet sinking unexpectedly into the sand are clues to back up and take another route.

*(continued )*

## Ghost shrimp–gray whales love 'em continued

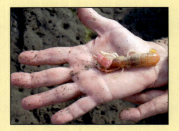

The pinkish ghost shrimp are beloved of gray whales that come into shallow Island County waters to scoop up bathtub-sized mouthfuls of muddy sand. They use their tongue and baleen to sieve out a feast of ghost shrimp.

These ghost shrimp beaches are found on the east side of Whidbey Island and on all sides of Camano Island. At low tide, the shallow hollows filled with water show where gray whales have fed.

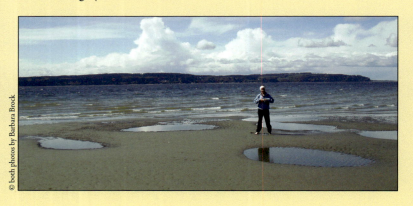

© both photos by Barbara Brock

| Site 50 | SOUTH WHIDBEY HARBOR AT LANGLEY |
|---------|----------------------------------|

### SOUTH WHIDBEY HARBOR AT LANGLEY
Lat/Long: 48.0383, -122.4039
228 Wharf Street, Langley

**Directions:** Located at the E end of downtown Langley off First St. Turn N onto Wharf St near the intersection of First and Second streets and follow signs down short hill and R to city dock and Phil Simon Park.

**Parking:** 10 👥 🚻 ⚓ ⛴ 🛶 🐚 🦀 🎣 🏠

**Adjoining public tideland:** 200 feet.

The floating docks at South Whidbey Harbor are open to the public from 9:00 a.m. to 9:00 p.m. An elevated fishing pier can be reached by the harbor access bridge. Enjoy a view across Saratoga Passage to Camano Island and east to the Cascades.

Sea stars, jellyfish, and crabs are visible from the dock and it's not unusual to see whales from shore. The beach is composed of sand and gravel and supports eelgrass beds in some of the lower tidal zones. This site is popular with scuba divers and kayakers.

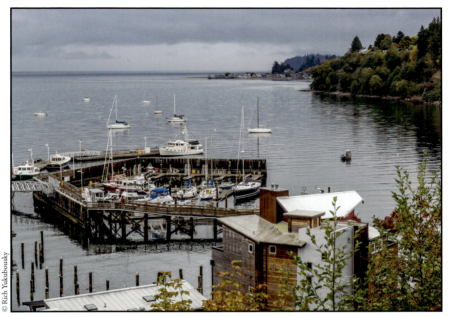

© Rich Yukubousky

*South Whidbey Harbor at Langley*

| Site 51 | MAXWELTON NATURE PRESERVE & OUTDOOR CLASSROOM (Fresh water) 7015 South Maxwelton Rd, Clinton |
|---|---|

**Directions:** From Hwy 525, turn S onto Maxwelton Rd and travel 3.5 miles to parking entrance on L, just before French Rd. A carved log salmon sculpture marks the site.

**Parking:** 7 🚶

This 6.75 acre preserve on Maxwelton Creek offers a self-guided interpretive trail, wetland boardwalk, and streamside viewing platforms. No dogs, please. Owned by South Whidbey School District, the preserve sits in a forested wetland of water-loving plants and sponge-like soils. A fully-equipped outdoor classroom, built with volunteer labor and community donations, is used by Whidbey Watershed Stewards both to educate hundreds of local students each year and to provide periodic classes for the community to learn about watersheds, habitat, and salmon.

There is no beach access at this site, but you are encouraged to enjoy the interpretive trail and surrounding natural spaces designated for public use. This is a beautiful site that highlights what south Whidbey's land- and fresh water-based ecosystems contribute to salmon populations and the health of local beaches.

## Whidbey's largest watershed

Maxwelton Creek was one of only two salmon-bearing streams on Whidbey Island, supporting coho (silver salmon) and sea-run cutthroat. The watershed extends north past the intermediate and high schools, and south to Swede Hill Road. The creek and its tributaries, such as Quade Creek, drain the watershed through more than 12 miles of streams before reaching the outflow at Maxwelton Beach, opposite the pond, where it runs under the road through a culvert and a tide gate. This tide gate prevents most salmon from entering the Maxwelton Creek system. Maxwelton Creek's brown cola color comes from the infusion of tannins as water flows through peat bogs on its way to Useless Bay.

At 7,834 acres, Maxwelton Watershed is the largest of 125 water-sheds in the county. The soil holds water year-round, slowing floods during winter rains and seeping moisture during dry summers. Native plants such as sword fern, salal, huckleberry, oceanspray, and Oregon grape help prevent erosion along stream banks.

In the 1990s, community volunteers came together to form the non-profit Maxwelton Salmon Adventure, which is now Whidbey Watershed Stewards. The Watershed Stewards run the Outdoor Classroom program for educating school children from public and private schools on Whidbey Island and beyond; they also work with the community to promote watershed stewardship and with interested landowners to restore and protect habitat on their creekside properties.

| **Site 52** | **DAVE MACKIE PARK** (Maxwelton Beach) |
| --- | --- |
| | Lat/Long: 47.9393, -122.4446 |
| | 7472 Maxwelton Rd, Clinton |

**Directions:** From Hwy 525, turn S onto Maxwelton Rd and travel 5 miles to the Maxwelton Beach community. The shoreside county park is on the R with 2 parking areas on either side of the ballfield.

**Parking:** 66 spaces; 9 of them are ADA parking spots.

**Adjoining public tideland:** 420 feet.

A popular family park with a ballfield, basketball hoop, play equipment, tables, benches, shelters, shower and dog wash, and sand beach. The site is co-owned by Island County and the Port of South Whidbey. Contact Island County Parks to reserve the group picnic shelter.

The tidelands are long and shallow, which may allow for some great tide-pooling opportunities but has also resulted in the closing of the boat ramp. For updates on the ramp closure search online for "Dave Mackie Park Island County."

There are beautiful views of Double Bluff and Useless Bay at this site. From fall to spring, many water birds feed in the bay between here and Double Bluff, including loons, grebes, ducks, and gulls. Brant geese stop by to browse on eelgrass. Driftwood and large woody debris may block stairs or access to amenities. The sand can be challenging for beach goers with mobility issues, so proceed with caution.

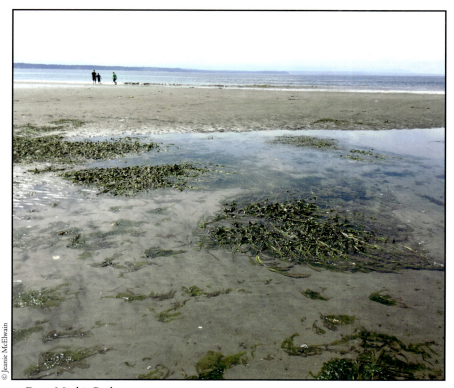

© Jeanie McElwain

*Dave Mackie Park*

## Maxwelton and the Chautauqua

For a few brief years in the early 1900s, tiny Maxwelton made a big name for itself. Situated below a 200-acre estuary formed by Island County's largest creek and watershed, Maxwelton hosted the first Northwest Chautauqua in 1910, attracting shiploads of summer visitors from throughout the Puget Sound region. The Chautauqua movement brought together social and religious interests, offering Bible study, recreation, and lectures on history, art, and science.

Four Scottish immigrant brothers had founded Maxwelton in 1905: Theodore Seaman Mackie, Peter Howard Mackie, David Thomas Mackie, and James Herbert Mackie. They promoted the Chautauqua by constructing an amphitheater to seat 4,000 and promising visitors a bathing beach with a quarter mile of clean white sand and ample tent sites. The Maxwelton Chautauqua ended in 1916 when heavy snows collapsed the amphitheater roof.

Today, Maxwelton is a quiet beach community of seasonal and year-round homes. Visitors picnic and play at Dave Mackie Park and walk the sandy beach. Every summer for a few hours, thousands of visitors still converge on Maxwelton for a community Fourth of July parade of several blocks that has become a Whidbey Island institution.

---

**Site 53**    **DEER LAKE PARK** (Fresh water)
4330 Bucktail Ln, Clinton

**Directions:** *a) From Hwy 525,* turn S onto Cultus Bay Rd. In 1.5 miles, turn L Deer Lake Rd. In 0.8 miles, go L to stay on Deer Lake Rd. In 0.4 miles, turn L onto Lake Shore Dr, then immediate L on Bucktail Ln. Park on either side of the lane and walk to the lake. *b) From Clinton Ferry,* turn L by Post Office onto Deer Lake Rd. In 1.2 miles, turn R onto Lake Shore Dr, then immediate L on Bucktail Ln.

**Parking:** 6 🛶 🪑 🏊 🏊 🐟

This lake is popular with families, paddlers, distance swimmers, and fishermen. At one end, there is a floating dock with a swimmers' ladder located inside a roped family swimming area. For fishing information, search online for "WDFW Fish Island Co Deer Lake." The access is owned by WDFW and managed by South Whidbey Parks and Recreation. There are many restrictions regarding the operation of motorized boats on the lake. See signs posted along Bucktail Lane for a list.

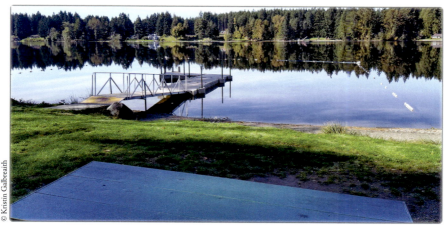

*Deer Lake swimming area*

## Site 54

### CLINTON BEACH & PIER
Lat/Long: 47.9752, -122.3515
6489 Hunziker Ln, Clinton

**Directions:** Located at the Clinton Ferry Terminal on the N side of the ferry dock. Turn N at the traffic light just before the ticket booths.

**Parking:** 6 spaces and 2 ADA spots for very limited, short-term parking. Public parking is available at the Port's lot on Humphrey Rd, the state park-and-ride lot at Deer Lake Rd, and the pay lot by the SE corner of the ferry dock.

ADA restroom and picnic tables.

**Adjoining public tideland:** 179 feet in front of the park.

Acquired by the Port of South Whidbey in 2004, this half-acre beachfront site is fully ADA accessible, including (in season) ADA mats that allow wheelchairs and walkers to get near water's edge. The picnic shelter features a living roof and a viewing platform made of recycled materials explained on interpretive signs.

Adjoining the site along the north side of the ferry dock is a public fishing pier and, beyond it, a ramp to a boat moorage dock (day use, 30-minutes or less). The beach is sandy, and eelgrass beds just offshore support a wide variety of life, including juvenile fish (see box pg. 29).

Although it's possible to launch a kayak or canoe, traveling south from here isn't recommended due to ferry traffic. North of the park is private beach; south of the park is the ferry dock. In season, the pier is used for crabbing and fishing. There's a cleaning sink, a shower-like washing station, a rinse station, a sand pile stocked with toys for children, and two large bronze sculptures. Large driftwood may accumulate and have to be crossed to reach the water's edge.

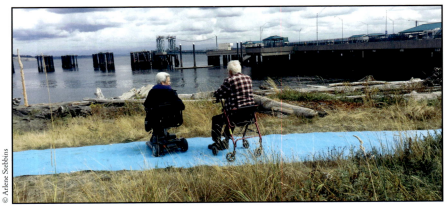

*Clinton Beach and Pier*

## Creosote-treated driftwood can be hazardous

Creosote, a coal tar by-product, has been found to pose serious health hazards to people and some aquatic life. Be aware that driftwood you find washed up on Puget Sound beaches may include creosote treated pieces and that handling them may pose a health risk. Also, burning creosoted wood in a campfire can cause harm if the smoke is inhaled. Chemicals in creosote leach into the environment and have been shown to cause damage to the eggs of small forage fish and other organisms that, as the foundation of the food web, are essential to salmon, birds, and other wildlife.

Creosote-impregnated wood smells like freshly poured asphalt and often oozes black tarry goo. The Washington Department of Natural Resources (WA DNR) has an ongoing program to identify and ultimately remove creosote logs from our coasts. Using a phone app called MyCoast, you can report creosote logs so that they can be located, removed, and properly disposed of by WA DNR. Go to **mycoast.org/wa.**

| Site 55 | GLENDALE BEACH PRESERVE |
|---|---|

**GLENDALE BEACH PRESERVE**
Lat/Long: 47.9385, -122.3582
Humphrey Rd and Glendale Rd, Clinton

**Directions:** From Hwy 525 uphill of the Clinton Ferry terminal, turn S onto Humphrey Rd. In 3 miles, at bottom of hill where road enters Glendale, continue straight to Glendale Beach gravel parking area on R.

**Parking:** 11 ⬛ 🏕 ⚓ 🐟 🛶 🏠

**Adjoining public tideland:** 420 feet.

Glendale Beach was protected in 2014 by the Whidbey Camano Land Trust. The mouth of Glendale Creek, one of only two salmon spawning creeks on Whidbey Island, is on the preserve. The property was once the terminus of the only railway ever to have existed in Island County, connecting Glendale to the Cultus Bay area, and was once a stop for the Mosquito Fleet ferry. The Glendale Hotel, built in 1911, stood here for over 100 years.

Mid-20th century, the creek was diverted into a concrete culvert, and unfortunately the structure prevented salmon from returning to spawn. Storms during the winter of 1996/1997 blew out the culvert, opening it to daylight. In the fall of 1997, after a 50-year absence, salmon returned to the lower reach of Glendale Creek. The county designed shorter crossing culverts and restored the lower channel, creating fish-friendly access above Glencale Road. Today the creek supports small spawning populations of chum and coho salmon.

Along the beachfront, the Whidbey Camano Land Trust worked with WA Department of Natural Resources to remove a creosote-treated bulkhead and pier to remove toxins, restore natural processes, and enhance habitat for salmon and other nearshore species.

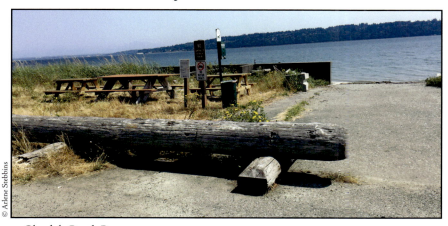

© Arlene Stebbins

*Glendale Beach Preserve*

| Site 56 | **POSSESSION POINT STATE PARK** |
|---------|---------------------------------|
|         | Lat/Long: 47.9075, -122.3765    |
|         | End of S Franklin Rd, Clinton   |

**Directions:** From Hwy 525, turn S at traffic light onto Cultus Bay Rd. In 4.7 miles, continue straight on Possession Rd, then in 0.2 mile, follow Possession Rd to R. Travel 1.3 miles and turn R onto S Franklin Rd. After 0.4 mile, a narrow parking area signals end of public road (no turning space for trailers). Follow beach trail leading down from parking area.

**Parking:** 10 🅿 🍴 🚶 🚤 🐟 🚶

**Adjoining public tideland:** None to north, nearly a mile south around Possession Point.

Possession Point is located on the far south end of Whidbey Island. This 25-acre park offers scenic beach walking around the bluff to the south where frequent slides continually reveal new geological stories. The park offers great opportunities for sightings of pigeon guillemots, kingfishers, herons, and bald eagles.

At the north end of the beach, there are three Cascadia Marine Trail campsites for specific use of campers in non-motorized boats.

The house is occupied by park staff; please respect their privacy.

For an upland trail to a high overlook, see page 183.

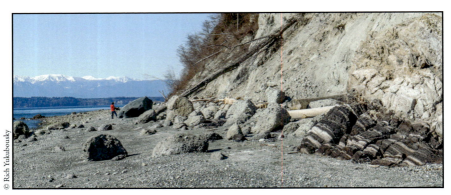

© Rich Yukubousky

*Possession Point State Park*

## Captain Vancouver was feeling possessive

Captain George Vancouver used Possession to name the shores he'd explored and claimed for the King. The ceremony took place on the east shore of Possession Sound, the body of water, 3-6 nautical miles wide and 9 nautical miles long, between the southern part of Whidbey Island and the mainland. It forms the entrance to Port Susan.

The Mukilteo-Clinton ferry crosses Possession Sound.

<table>
<tr><td>**Site 57**</td><td>**POSSESSION BEACH WATERFRONT PARK**</td></tr>
</table>

## POSSESSION BEACH WATERFRONT PARK

Lat/Long: 47.9121, -122.3757

8212 Possession Rd, Clinton

**Directions:** From Hwy 525, turn S on Cultus Bay Rd. In 4.7 miles, continue straight on Possession Rd, then in 0.2 mile, follow Possession Rd to R. Travel 1.3 miles, and 50 feet past S Franklin Rd, turn R into entry road to park and boat launch.

**Parking:** 30 total spaces; 19 are for trailered vehicles. Paved sidewalk leads from parking area downhill to boat launch. Overnight parking is available for a fee, and permits may be purchased at park kiosk. Note that the park is open from dawn to dusk and vehicles may be accessed only when the park is open.

Dock floats are seasonal.

**Adjoining public tideland:** 677 feet.

This day-use park and launch gives access to one of the most superb sport fishing areas in Puget Sound. Anglers can catch their limits of lingcod during bottom fish openings. Several species of salmon run off the point during migration and are a prize during seasonal openings.

This site offers a fine view of the ferries plying back and forth between Clinton and Mukilteo as well as the busy boat traffic in Possession Sound. It's also common to see a variety of wildlife from shore, including deer, bald eagles, whales, seals, and sea lions. The view is enhanced by taking the Dorothy Cleveland Trail, a 1½ mile round trip walk uphill to an elevation of 390 feet.

The boat ramp was refurbished in 2017. Be aware that the floats are removed during the winter season. A webcam offers live video of the boat launch. Camping is prohibited.

The park is owned by the Port of South Whidbey. For more information search online for Possession Beach Waterfront Park.

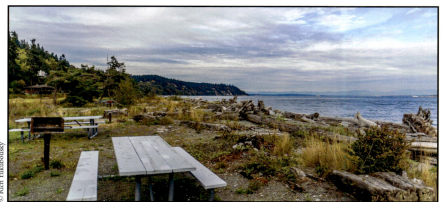

© Rich Yukubousky

*Possession Beach Waterfront Park*

# Derelict gear keeps on killing

Out of sight and out of mind, a tragic waste occurs every day in waters surrounding us—and beyond. Salmon, shellfish, bottom fish, marine mammals, aquatic birds, and other creatures fall victim to thousands of lost commercial fishing nets, crab pots, shrimp pots, discarded lines, and recreational gear. For example, the over 12,000 crab pots lost yearly in Puget Sound kill an estimated 180,000 crabs in addition to creatures who enter the pots to eat the dead trapped crabs.

Humans, too, fall victim to derelict debris. Both divers and swimmers become entangled in the nets and lines. Lost gear also wraps around the rudders and propellers of recreational and commercial vessels, potentially endangering the crews.

Trained dive crews have removed more than 5,800 derelict fishing nets from Puget Sound. Removal of these nets is estimated to save over 400 marine mammals, birds, and fish each day. The Marine Resource Committees and Northwest Straits Initiative continue to lead the work in preventing and removing derelict gear in Puget Sound.

Report the discovery of derelict gear, whether in the water or on shore, to the Washington Department of Fish & Wildlife. There are no penalties for reporting lost fishing gear. Other hazards—such as 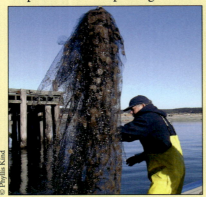 abandoned boats, large marine debris, and creosote debris—can be reported through an app at **mycoast.org/wa.** If you find a live animal caught in any kind of entanglement, immediately call the Marine Entanglements Hotline at 877-767-9425. Dead entangled animals should be reported at the same number.

*A derelict fishing net is hoisted from the waters off Keystone Spit on west Whidbey Island. An experienced crew from Natural Resources Consultants cut the net free and removed it as part of a cleanup project for the Northwest Straits Commission and Island County Marine Resources Committee. The net had been snagged on pilings at this popular diving location for more than a year, posing a hazard to scuba divers and killing marine life entangled in it. The dock where it was snagged is a nesting site for pigeon guillemots and a roost for cormorants.*

© Phyllis Kind

# CAMANO ISLAND SITES

Sixteen miles long and from one to seven miles wide, Camano Island is tucked between Whidbey Island to the west and the mainland to the east. It's surrounded by the waters of Port Susan, Skagit Bay, and Saratoga Passage.

Camano Island is connected to the mainland at Stanwood by the Camano Gateway bridge. From the bridge, Hwy 532 continues three miles west to a directory for the island located at Terry's Corner. Here the road splits, with East Camano Drive to the left and North Camano Drive to the right. Terry's Corner is the reference point for directions to Camano Island sites listed in this book.

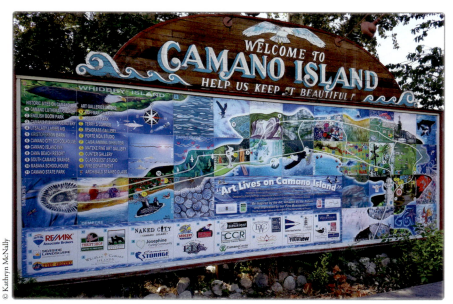

*Terry's Corner landmark sign, Camano Island*

© Kathryn McNally

| Site 58 | ENGLISH BOOM HISTORICAL PRESERVE |
|---|---|
| | Lat/Long: 48.2626, -122.4385 |
| | End of Moore Rd, Camano Island |

**Directions:** *a) From Hwy 532,* turn N onto Good Rd (about 2 miles E of Terry's Corner or 1 mile W of Camano Gateway Bridge). Continue 1.9 miles as road turns W and becomes Utsalady Rd. Just past Camano Island Airfield, turn N onto Moore Rd and drive 0.6 mile to road end. *b) From Terry's Corner,* drive W 1.1 miles on North Camano Dr, turn R on Arrowhead Rd, drive 0.2

miles N to Utsalady Rd, turn R onto Utsalady and travel 1.4 miles E, turning N onto Moore Rd and driving 0.6 mile to road end.

**Parking:** 6 cars, 2 ADA. 8 more spaces on right 0.1 mile uphill from road-end parking area. 🎏 🏠 🛬 🐦 🚶 ⛺

**Adjoining public tideland:** 300 feet with trail easement to east across private land.

In clear weather, this site has spectacular views of Mount Baker and the Cascades. The history of logging days at English Boom is told at a kiosk. The site has 60 feet of ADA-accessible boardwalk for wildlife viewing, another trail through salt marsh to the end of the property and continuing on an easement, and over 500 acres of salt marsh, mudflat, and beach berm on the shore of Skagit Bay, offering habitat for waterfowl, shorebirds, and raptors. Island County owns seven acres near the west end of this area.

Decaying pilings, reminders of a once extensive log storage system, provide perches for fish-hunting birds such as bald eagles, ospreys, herons, and kingfishers. Birdhouses have been erected for purple martins, the largest North American swallow. An active eagle's nest can be viewed from the parking area.

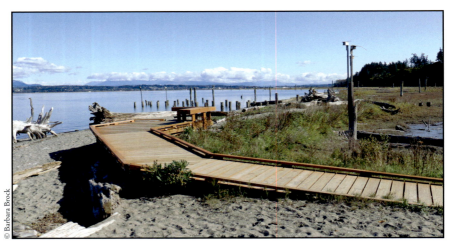

*English Boom Historical Preserve*

## Ospreys carry their catch aerodynamically

Ospreys are the only North American raptors that feed exclusively on fish.

These birds migrate in the fall, some traveling as far south as Central America. They return in mid-April to build large stick platform nests in treetops or on high platforms. Ospreys also nest on channel markers in harbors and on a wide array of artificial sites, selecting locations where fishing is good.

Because these fishers can access only the top two or three feet of water, they look for surface-schooling fish or shallow water. When an osprey spies its prey, it stretches both legs in front and dives toward the water. As it grasps a fish with its sharp talons, it flies on without landing as it maneuvers the fish head first into an aerodynamic flight position for the trip back to the nest.

## Great blue herons spear their food

With its long neck and legs, the great blue heron is a familiar sight standing sentinel on docks, hunkered on the mudflats, or wading in shallow water.

When feeding, the great blue heron stands motionless in knee-deep water watching for fish, its long neck recoiled. Then in a surge of power, the bird jabs its sharp bill into the water to spear a fish. If successful, the heron shuffles the fish into its beak and swallows it whole. Taking a few more steps, the heron pauses and again assumes a hunting stance, eyes focused into the water.

Here in the Pacific Northwest, this adaptive species also stalks pastures and roadsides, hunting small mammals, reptiles, amphibians, and insects.

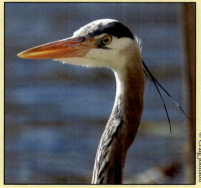

© Craig Johnson

## Site 59 — UTSALADY BEACH

Lat/Long: 48.2538, -122.4983

End of Utsalady Point Rd, Camano Island

**Directions:** From Terry's Corner, follow North Camano Dr 2.9 miles. Turn N onto Utsalady Point Rd. Keep to R and proceed downhill 0.25 mile to parking area and boat launch.

**Parking:** 10. Boat launch fee: Pay daily pass onsite or online at Island County website (annual pass also available): **islandcountywa.gov/PublicWorks/Parks.**

**Adjoining public tideland:** 380 feet.

This access has a single lane concrete boat ramp. Loaner life jackets are available. Beyond the parking lot is a grassy area with picnic tables; enjoy scenic views of the Cascades, Skagit Bay, and Whidbey Island. Smelting is a popular activity.

Today Utsalady Bay is home to beachside houses and moored pleasure boats, but in the late 1800s it was home to a large sawmill and a working port with sailing ships carrying lumber to world markets. Utsalady also served as a landing for the ferry between Camano and Whidbey Island (see box pgs. 40-41). This access has close neighbors; please respect private property and do not park along the road.

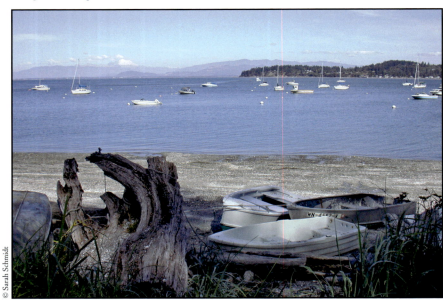

*Utsalady Beach*

# Utsalady Bay

At one time Skagit Bay, at the mouth of the South Fork of the Skagit River and just north of Camano's Utsalady Bay, was the richest herring ground in all the Salish Sea. The herring spawn in spring attracts whales, sea lions, eagles, and people. Coast Salish tribes used the landing on the north end of Camano Island continuously for thousands of years before settlers arrived.

Salmon began their upriver trek at the mouth of the Skagit. In the 1850s, settlers were quick to discover the merits of Utsalady Bay, including shelter from storms that blow from the southeast.

A sawmill ran from 1858 through 1890 to handle timber from logjams on the Skagit River and trees harvested from Camano and northern Puget Sound. Abandoned pilings from the shipping dock remain at Utsalady Beach Park. The mill became a hub on north Camano Island where a ferry ran from Whidbey Island.

Utsalady Ladies' Aid was founded in 1908 to serve the growing needs of the community and improve quality of life for the families. Their historic 1923 building still stands and the organization remains very active.

## Site 60 — UTSALADY VISTA PARK
398 Shore Dr, Camano Island

**Directions:** From Terry's Corner, follow North Camano Dr for 3 miles. Turn N on Utsalady Point Rd. The vista point and parking are directly ahead on L.

**Parking:** 4

This grassy pocket park atop the bluff at Utsalady Point is a county historic site featuring picnic tables, a view over Utsalady Bay and toward Mount Baker, and a carved bas-relief historical marker depicting the sawmill era. There is no access to the beach.

## Site 61 — MAPLE GROVE PARK
Lat/Long: 48.2528, -122.5177
Boat Ramp Rd, Camano Island

**Directions:** From Terry's Corner, follow North Camano Dr 3.1 miles and take a lazy R turn onto Maple Grove Rd. Drive 0.5 mile to boat ramp and parking on the R.

**Parking:** 6 plus 12 spaces for vehicles with boat trailers. Boat launch fee: pay daily pass onsite, or daily or annual pass online (see Site 59).

⬛ 🏕 ⬛ 🦅

**Adjoining public tideland:** 250 feet in front and west of boat launch.

The rocky shores of Maple Grove offer access to the Skagit estuary and the north end of Saratoga Passage. Enjoy views of Whidbey Island, Skagit Bay, and the Cascades. Cormorants can often be seen on the pilings, drying their wings after a dive for fish. Smelt spawn on the high tide in this area. The county boat launch can be very busy during the height of crabbing season. This access has close neighbors; please respect private property and park only in the designated area.

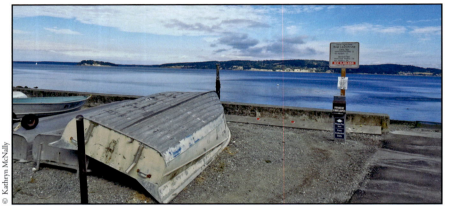

Maple Grove Park

## Camano Island–A Community Wildlife Habitat

Camano Island enjoys a rare distinction: the entire island was the 10th community in the nation certified by the National Wildlife Federation (NWF) as a Community Wildlife Habitat. Certification was in 2005 with 500 properties; many more have since been added, and the goal is to reach 1,000. As single- and multi-family residences, businesses, schools, community areas, shorelines, and demonstration gardens individually certify their yards and gardens as wildlife habitats, island residents create safe wildlife corridors, as well as clean water resources.

*(continued)*

## Camano Island—wildlife habitat continued

A wildlife habitat requires five essential elements, either present naturally or provided by the homeowner: food, water, shelter/cover, place to raise a family, and sustainable garden practices. Sustainable gardening techniques improve the health of the soil, air, water, and habitat for all.

Islanders have become visible members of a network of thousands of people in the nation who share their living spaces—ranging in size from a small deck to acres of land—with wildlife.

Applications and help are available from Friends of Camano Island Parks (FOCIP): **camanowildlifehabitat@gmail.com** and **camanowildlifehabitat.org.** Wildlife Habitat certification is through the NWF: **nwf.org.** A small fee is charged for processing; members receive a certificate, the NWF "Habitats" newsletter, and a one-year subscription to National Wildlife Magazine.

**Site 62**

### LIVINGSTON BAY (Fox Trot Way)
Lat/Long: 48.2366, -122.4337
End of Fox Trot Way, Camano Island

**Directions:** From Terry's Corner, travel 1 mile E on Hwy 532  Turn S onto Fox Trot Way and proceed straight 0.2 mile to the road end access.

**Parking:** 10-15

**Adjoining public tideland:** 90 feet (road width).

Livingston Bay is a critical stop on the Pacific flyway for waterfowl and other migratory birds and provides vital estuarine rearing habitat for sturgeon, salmon, steelhead, cutthroat, and other fish species, as well as gray whales. The Whidbey Camano Land Trust permanently protected 3,218 acres of tidelands in the bay in 2006, in part to ensure effective management of Port Susan Bay, a Western Shorebird Site of Regional Importance. In 2008 there was a large effort here to remove Spartina, an exotic weed that harms tidelands (see box pg. 39).

A mudflat at lower tides, Livingston can be used by shallow draft boats, canoes, or kayaks only during the high tides. If you're caught in the bay in anything less than a high tide, you will certainly be like a fish out of water.

A broad expanse of driftwood separates road end and tideland.

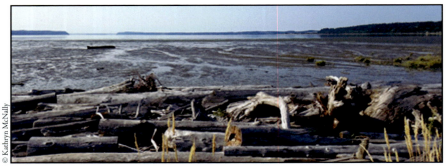

*Livingston Bay view*

## Pocket estuaries–Island County's salmon nurseries

Whidbey and Camano Islands don't have major rivers, but the islands are at the confluence of three major rivers on the mainland: the Skagit, Stillaguamish, and Snohomish. Endangered Chinook, as well as coho and chum salmon, spawn in these rivers. After the eggs hatch, the young salmon fry (about two inches long) rely heavily on the shallow, nutrient-rich waters along Whidbey and Camano Island shores to feed and grow before heading out to sea. Areas within five miles (one tidal exchange) of the mouths of the rivers are especially important, including the northeastern shore of Whidbey Island and the north and eastern shores of Camano Island.

Early studies focused on salmonid use of pocket estuaries–small, partially-enclosed marshy areas where fresh water outflows dilute the sea's normal salinity. This environment is rich with a diversity of plants and insects, and tidal action is moderated. Examples of pocket estuaries include Triangle Cove and Elger Bay on Camano Island and also Ala Spit and Cornet Bay on Whidbey Island.

Early seining studies were expanded to include studies of salmonid use of small streams in the Whidbey Basin, which showed their importance as rearing habitat. That resulted in increased efforts to improve the streams' connectivity to salt water by replacing culverts and tide gates that block fish from getting upstream (see box pgs. 112-113). Studies have shown the nearshore also provides nursery habitat for forage fish, which are an important food source for adult salmon.

*(continued)*

## Pocket estuaries continued

The nearshore is heavily influenced by feeder bluffs and the tidal drift that distributes sand and gravel. A priority for salmon recovery is conserving and restoring these features as well as reducing shoreline armoring where possible and encouraging the use of soft-shore stabilization (see box pgs. 25-26). These measures also help the health of important eelgrass beds (see box pg. 29) and other links in the food web.

Recently, the impacts of climate change and sea level rise have been incorporated into salmon recovery strategies to encourage responsible actions leading to resilient habitats. For more information, search for Salmon Recovery Plan on the Island County website.

## Site 63

### IVERSON SPIT PRESERVE
Lat/Long: 48.2115, -122.4419
End of Iverson Rd, Camano Island

**Directions:** *(a) From Terry's Corner*, travel S on East Camano Dr for 2.7 miles to Russell Rd. Turn L, go 1 mile E on Russell Rd, turn R onto Sunrise Blvd for 0.2 mile, then L onto Iverson Beach Rd for 0.5 mile (L at T and down steep hill) to stop sign, then L onto Iverson Rd for 0.5 mile to road end. *(b) From Terry's Corner traffic light*, turn S onto Sunrise Blvd for 2.5 miles, turn L onto Iverson Beach Rd and continue as above. (Just 0.2 mile further on Sunrise Blvd is Barnum Point, Site 68.)

**Parking:** 10 in the lot; additional parking is in adjoining county-owned field.

**Adjoining public tideland:** None to south, 2,400 feet north to end of spit.

This mixture of marsh and farm fields at the southwest corner of Livingston Bay, historically a tidal salt marsh, was diked for farming in the 1940s. The 120-acre property was acquired by Island County in 1999 with Conservation Futures funding. A 1-mile loop trail takes the walker through wetland, thickets, lowland forest and field edges. Over 125 bird species have been recorded here.

A boardwalk, with viewing platforms and boxed steps over the dike, has been added to reduce erosion. The beach beyond a wide expanse of drift logs offers views of both Mount Baker and Mount Rainier. Be mindful that logs may be blocking parts of the path, and you may need to take a longer path to the beach. Tides at this location move quickly and can trap beachgoers who venture too far onto the sand flats. Always be aware of low and high tide times and stay close to shore.

Interpretive signs about the local wildlife and marine ecology are a great opportunity to learn how you can leave a positive impact.

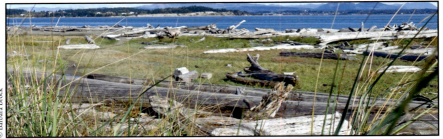

*Iverson Spit Preserve*

## Kristoferson Creek- Camano Island's largest salmon stream

Tucked inside a sheltered right-angle bend on Camano Island's inside east shore is Triangle Cove, a 200-acre pocket estuary at the mouth of Kristoferson Creek (see box previous two pages). The creek drains the island's second largest watershed and is its largest salmon stream. Scientists have documented Kristoferson Creek as one of the important small streams for salmonids in the Whidbey Basin.

Three species of salmon, at three different life stages, use the creek. There's a small run of adult chum, 30-plus inches, that spawn each fall in the stream gravels above Russell Road. Coho juveniles (smolt), about four inches, are noted for rearing in beaver marsh habitat, such as above East Camano Drive/Can Ku Road, then migrating with spring runoff down to the salt water. Chinook juveniles (fry), approximately two inches, use the lower reaches of the creek as important rearing habitat in the spring.

Kristoferson Creek is not a Chinook spawning stream, but fry from nearby rivers, such as the Stillaguamish, Skagit, and even the Snohomish have been documented using the lower reaches of Kristoferson Creek. The mixing of the fresh and salt water give the fish a chance to adjust to the saltwater environment and grow in size before heading to the ocean. A larger size generally results in a greater survival rate.

Recently, partially-blocking culverts (Photo A, next page) were replaced with fish-friendly culverts (Photo B, next page) under two Island County roads on the lower portion of Kristoferson Creek.

*(continued)*

# Kristoferson Creek continued

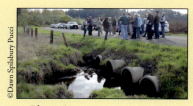
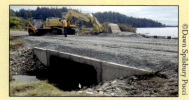

Photo A                                   Photo B

Planning is underway for replacement of other fish-blocking culverts in the watershed, both by Island County and by private landowners. The goal is to allow fish access to the entire main channel of the creek.

In 2005, Conservation Futures funding was used to acquire 2.5 acres and nearly 255 feet along both sides on the lower reach of the creek above Russell Road. Managed by Island County Parks as Kristoferson Creek Habitat, this provides a publicly owned location with access to the creek for education and wildlife viewing. Friends of Camano Island Parks (FOCIP) built and maintains a short trail system with a viewing platform and bridge at the creek. A second rustic viewing site and bench is located at the "Cedar Grove," about 100 feet upstream of the bridge. An additional 7.5 acres of property downstream, including 520 feet of creek, were protected in 2008 by the Whidbey Camano Land Trust so that 10 acres are now preserved along Kristoferson Creek.

Farther upstream in the Kristoferson/Triangle watershed is an extensive beaver marsh. Much of it is privately owned, but there is public access at two points along Can Ku Road, across from the animal shelter. One-half block west of East Camano Dr, there's a short trail to a viewing platform, which looks out over the lower part of the marsh. Right at the intersection of Can Ku Road and East Camano Dr, a trail leads to the "Beaver Deceiver," a water leveling device installed by Island County at the outlet of the beaver marsh to manage the water level to protect downstream properties while allowing beavers to maintain their habitat. Beaver marsh habitat is important for flood control and water quality as well as providing rearing habitat for juvenile coho.

*Driving directions to Kristoferson Creek Habitat: From Terry's Corner, follow East Camano Dr S for 2 miles; turn L onto Russell Rd. After a long block, turn L onto Sapphire Dr. The first cross street is David St; just before you reach it, on L you will see a field with a small sign. Park on the road shoulder. The short trail leads to an informational kiosk, bridge, and viewing platform. From the kiosk, there is also a short trail to "Cedar Grove." Trail mileage is under 0.5 mile.*

## CAVALERO PARK

Lat/Long: 48.1744, -122.4773
1013 Simonsen Place, Camano Island

**Directions:** From Terry's Corner, follow East Camano Dr 5.5 miles. Turn E onto Cavalero Rd and in 0.25 mile, follow the signs to the L onto a narrow, steep, winding single-lane road that drops down to the park.

**Parking:** 15-20, including spaces to accommodate boat trailers. Boat launch fee site: Pay daily pass onsite or daily and annual pass online at Island County website (See Site 59). 🚻 ⛱ 🛶 🛫 ⚓ 🅿

**Adjoining public tideland:** 250 feet at park.

This rocky shore gives way to a shallow sandy tideland at the lower tides, making it a popular swimming area. Cavalero Park is the only public launch on Camano Island's Port Susan side. The boat ramp, usable only at high tide, is not appropriate for launching large boats due to the steep, single lane access road. Loaner life jackets are available.

The site offers a scenic panorama from Mount Baker to Three Fingers mountain. Look for great blue herons roosting in trees along the bluff to the north or feeding in the bay at low tide. Be aware that there is private property located on either side of the public beach; please be courteous.

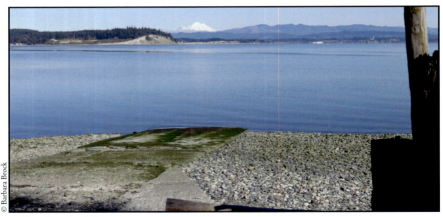

© Barbara Brock

*Cavalero Park boat ramp*

## CAMA BEACH HISTORICAL STATE PARK

Site 65

Lat/Long: 48.1409, -122.5147
1880 West Camano Dr, Camano Island

**Directions:** From Terry's Corner, go S on East Camano Dr about 6 miles. When East Camano Dr heads L, keep R on main road, now Elger Bay Rd. At

Elger Bay Grocery and gas station, turn W onto Mountain View Rd (becomes West Camano Dr). Go 2.5 miles up a steep hill, then follow West Camano Dr to the R and look for park entrance on L.

**Parking:** Plentiful. A Discover Pass is required to park here.

🚻 🚗 🪧 🚶 🛶 🐟 ⛵ 🥾

**Adjoining public tideland:** Approximately 1.1 miles.

Cama Beach is 463 acres with 6,000 feet of pebbled/sandy beach. The park has a five-acre lake, a dense second growth forest, three miles of trails, and a one-mile trail connecting to Camano Island State Park.

The site has experienced four human histories: Coast Salish people for thousands of years until 1855; a logging camp from the 1850s to 1906; an auto court resort from 1932 until 1989; and a state park from 2008 until today. Recognized for the collection of buildings, this Depression Era auto court is the only one of its kind on the National Register of Historic Places.

The park has 50 historic buildings, 34 cabins rented out to the public (reservations required), an historic store operated by the Cama Beach Foundation, rowboats and kayaks for rent by the Center for Wooden Boats, and a restaurant operated by the Cama Café located in the Cama Center. Cama Center is available for special events such as weddings or meetings.

There are fun and educational activities at the park year-round, sponsored by Cama Beach Foundation, Sound Water Stewards, and other partners as listed on the Cama Beach Foundation website.

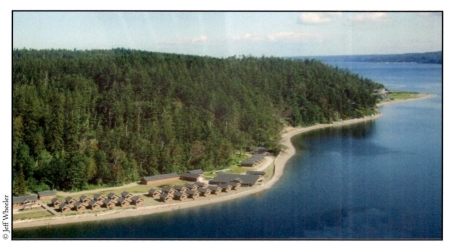

*Aerial view of Cama Beach State Park*

## What's in a name?

### Camano

Camano Island is named for Lt. Don Jacinto Caamano of the Spanish Navy who, during the 1700s, had explored as far north as Alaska from the Spanish naval base in San Blas, Mexico. However, Caamano never entered Puget Sound. The island's name was given in 1847 by a British surveyor as part of an effort to restore Spanish names in the area.

The local Salish called it *Kol-lut-chen,* "land jutting out into a bay."

### Port Susan

While charting the waters searching for the Northwest Passage in 1792, Captain George Vancouver got both *HMS Discovery* and *HMS Chatham* stuck in the mud of the waters of Port Susan during low tides typical of that area. The sailors who allowed the *Chatham* to go aground were flogged.

Vancouver later named Port Susan after the highly respected Lord Admiral Alan Gardner's wife. Lady Susanna Gale Gardner was born to a wealthy family; her grandfather owned the only silver mine in Jamaica where Susanna was raised.

Vancouver was an accomplished cartographer in the British Navy and mapped the Pacific Coast from the Bering Strait to California. He named many other places after British citizens, including Puget Sound; Whidbey and Vashon Islands; and mountains Baker, Hood, Rainier, and St. Helens.

*[Resource: Stuck in the Mud, 2011, by Penny Hutchison Buse of Warm Beach]*

| **Site 66** | **CAMANO ISLAND STATE PARK** |
|---|---|
| | Lat/Long: boat ramp 48.1240, -122.4953, beach near restrooms 48.1211, -122.4912, and Marine Trail campsite 48.1209, -122.4905 |
| | 2269 Lowell Point Rd, Camano Island |

**Directions:** From Terry's Corner, go S on East Camano Dr about 6 miles. When East Camano Dr heads L, keep R on main road, which is now Elger Bay Rd. At Elger Bay Grocery and gas station, turn R onto Mountain View

Rd. Go 2 miles, up a steep hill, then turn L onto Lowell Point Rd and follow to park entrance.

**Parking**: 30 plus 25 for vehicles with boat trailers. A Discover Pass is required to park here; an additional permit is needed to use boat ramp.

**Adjoining Public Tideland:** 1.25 miles.

In the late 1940s, locals realized that public access to the water was almost gone. The South Camano Grange worked with Washington State Parks and the local population to build a park in one day. By the day's end, the volunteers had built picnic tables, cleared land and paths, and leveled a road and parking area. They had provided a place for everyone to get to the beach. All labor—3,561 person-hours and 376 machine hours—and all expenses had been donated. That day was July 27, 1949, and the park opened to the public the next day.

The original park is now the North Beach area; the Lowell Point section was added in the early 1960s. The park is now 244 acres in size with 6,700 feet of pebbled beach. Amenities include 77 wooded campsites plus a Marine Trail campsite; a group camp; six miles of bluff and forest trails including a one-mile trail connecting to Cama Beach State Park; an interpretive trail with 18 points of interest; a two-lane boat ramp with finger piers; two picnic shelters; 50+ picnic sites, many right on the beach; five rental cabins (reservations required); and an amphitheater with summer programs.

ADA accessible restrooms are at the Group Camp, main campground, North Beach parking area, and near the boat ramp.

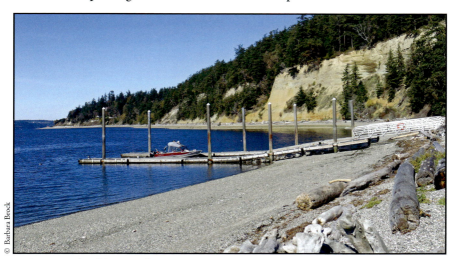

© Barbara Brock

*Camano Island State Park*

# At the beach with your dog

Many people love dogs, so much so that there are an estimated 90 million dogs in the U.S. People also love beaches, so putting the two together makes for a fabulous day enjoying the beach with your best friend. One challenge to this day of pleasure is dog waste.

You may ask, "What's the difference between local wildlife scat and that from my dog?"

The truth is twofold. First, local wildlife takes in nutrients from the local environment and then returns them as a new nutrient resource. However, our canine friends eat an extremely nutrient-rich diet. That nutrient load, often high in nitrogen and phosphorous, is not coming from the local environment but is adding to it. This isn't a healthy closed-loop system. Second, dogs carry high levels of bacteria and parasites that are harmful to the environment and wildlife. In both instances, the problem is compounded by a matter of scale both in the sheer number of dogs we love and the high degree of harm from their poop. A study by the National Institutes of Health on a Florida beach found that one dog fecal event was equal in dangerous microbial load to that of over 6,000 bird fecal events. Multiply that by hundreds of dog visitors.

*So what can we do to make playing with our dogs at the shore safer for the marine environment?*

- **When headed to the beach**, most dogs get excited and need to relieve themselves. Walk them around the parking lot or take them on a short trail near the beach before taking them to the water. Let them do their business, **bag it and place it in a receptacle or lay the bagged poop in your trunk to dispose of in the landfill.**
- **If you are already at the beach** and your pup just can't wait, be very sure to scoop the entire poop from the beach, bag it, and toss it in a receptacle or put the bagged poop in your trunk to dispose of in the landfill.
- **Never drop a plastic or "biodegradable" poop bag!** If you do drop the bag, the beach environment is degraded not only by microbial load from the poop, but also by the plastic debris.
- **If you reside at or near the beach,** be sure to scoop the poop in your yard as it occurs, or at least every other day. Don't let it sit and allow the microbial load to leach into the ground and end up in the water. Always send the bagged poop to the landfill.

*Love your pooch, love your beach, and protect them both.*

## Beach hoppers aren't fleas and don't bite

If you move aside a pile of washed up seaweed, chances are you'll see a flurry of wild, random hopping by hordes of minute creatures. These are beach hoppers, tiny crustaceans that stay just above the water level as it moves up and down with the tides.

Beach hoppers are sometimes called "sand fleas" but they're not fleas or even insects; they are crustaceans, related to shrimp. Nor do they bite. If you try to hold them in your hand, you may feel a sharp prickle. That's not their teeth but instead their feet, pointed to help them cling to the decomposing seaweed in which they feed and seek refuge.

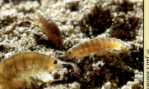

These tiny crustaceans eat decaying plant matter that washes up on the beach. In turn, they are eaten by many birds as well as insects and even raccoons.

© Jan Holmes

---

**Site 67**  ### TILLICUM BEACH
Lat/Long: 48.1036, -122.4000
2947 Tillicum Beach Dr, Camano Island

**Directions:** From Terry's Corner, follow East Camano Dr S for 11.7 miles. Turn E onto Karen Way and continue 0.4 mile to bottom of hill. Turn L on Tillicum Beach Dr to access on the water side with small parking area opposite.

**Parking:** 4 🏕 🚻

**Adjoining public tideland:** 80 feet of community beach dedicated to the public.

This pleasant and quiet pocket park in the middle of a small beachfront community provides a panoramic view of the Cascade Mountain Range. Please drive slowly and respect private property. Launching or landing a hand-carry boat may be difficult at high tide because of large quantities of driftwood sloshing against the shore. Driftwood may also make walking access difficult, so take caution at this site.

# When travel was an adventure

Early settlers traveled in style among local communities on the steamers *Camano* and *Whidby*, which carried passengers and freight daily from about 1906 to 1912. This was the era of the Mosquito Fleet of Puget Sound lore–the heyday of stern-wheelers, side-wheelers, and propeller-driven craft. This schedule appeared in The Camano Enterprise in 1907.

The steamers were built in Coupeville by Captain H. B. Lovejoy; both vessels were lost in separate accidents after just a few years, but others picked up the slack. The steamers filled a need: early roads were primitive; Camano Island finally acquired its bridge to the mainland in 1909, but Whidbey Island went without until 1935. Most Camano passengers used the Camano "City" dock near Chapman Creek, where a few remnants are still visible by the current Camano Island Inn. Before a dock was built at Mabana, passengers often rowed out to be picked up. The Whidbey stop called Saratoga was about four miles north of Langley.

## Island Transportation Co.

### Str. ,'Whidby" Time Card:

LEAVING

| NORTH BOUND | SOUTH BOUND |
|---|---|
| Seattle.........4 P. M. | LaConner (Subject to |
| (Except Sat. and Sun.' | tide) |
| Sun. 3 p. m. touching | Utsaladdy...6;30 A. M. |
| Everett.) | Oak Harbor 7:15 " |
| Clinton......6:15 P. M. | San de Fuca 7:45 " |
| Langley..... 6:45 " | Coupeville 8:30 " |
| Saratoga.....7:05 " | Camano.... 9:15 " |
| Camano......7:45 " | Saratoga....9:45 " |
| Coupeville...8:30 " | Langley....10:10 " |
| Oak Harbor...9:15 " | Clinton....10:35 " |
| | Arriv'g Seattle 1 P. M. |

### Str. "Camano" Time Card
(Daily except Sunday.)
LEAVING SOUTH BOUND

| Coupeville:........... .... ..........7:00 A. M. |
| Oak Harbor...................7:30 " |
| Camano ..... .. ...............8:15 " |
| Langley ............. .. .. .. 9:15 " |
| Clinton ............................ 9:45 " |
| Arriving at Everett...... .... ... 10:15 " |

Leaving Everett for Coupeville, 3 P. M.

Brown's Point, San de Fuca and Saratoga, subject to call.

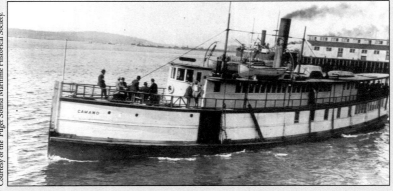

Courtesy of the Puget Sound Maritime Historical Society.

## BARNUM POINT COUNTY PARK

**Site 68**

Lat/Long: 48.1980, -122.4540
278 Sunrise Blvd, Camano Island

**Directions**: From Terry's Corner traffic light, turn S onto Sunrise Blvd for 2.7 miles to the Barnum Point County Park parking lot (just 0.2 mile past the turn to Iverson Spit, Site 63).

**Parking**: 19 in graveled lot; also room for school buses.

**Adjoining public tideland**: Approximately 1 mile.

Barnum Point County Park highlights the best of Camano Island's natural beauty, featuring mature coastal forest; sweeping views of the Cascade Mountains from Mount Baker to Mount Rainier; the waters of Port Susan from Kayak Point to South Camano around to Driftwood Shores and Triangle Cove; and more than a mile of unspoiled beach. The park is the result of cooperative efforts with many stakeholders, beginning as 27 acres expanded six-fold following the acquisition of six parcels between 2016-18, five of which are waterfront; now more than 7,000 acres of prime habitat are protected. This area is part of the Greater Skagit and Stillaguamish Delta, which is a Site of Regional Importance in the Western Hemisphere Shorebird Reserve Network. For a complete history and photos see: **wclt.org/projects/barnum-point/**.

The park features over 2.5 miles of groomed upland trails winding through mature forest, open meadows, and marsh. There are two pedestrian accesses to a mile of natural beach. One is about ½ mile down an old gravel driveway with a steep slope to the beach. The second access is approximately one mile from the parking lot to beach on nearly level trail. The beach between the two accesses is backed by high bluff, so walking between them should be planned with consideration for the tides.

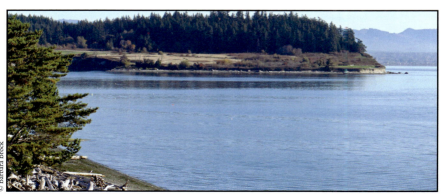

© Barbara Brock

*Barnum Point County Park*

# Beach plants are well worth a look

When you get to the beach, don't forget to look at the backshore plants. This vegetation grows high on the beach near the line marked by driftwood stranded during very high tides. Many of these plants serve an important role on the beach because their root systems help stabilize the sand.

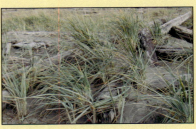

The native dunegrass (*Elymus mollis*), with blades more than three feet high and one-half inch wide, is blue-gray with a rather powdery texture. Dunegrass was used by indigenous peoples for weaving pack straps and baskets.

*Dunegrass*

Both American and European sea rocket (*Cakile edentula* and *C. maritima*) are mustard family annuals inhabiting Island County beaches. Sea rocket is a pioneer species, among the first to move into areas of barren sandy dunes, and has unique seed pods that pop apart into two sections when mature. One section remains attached to the parent plant, to be buried by blowing sand and then to bring new growth in the same place the following season. The other section floats away with the tides to colonize new territory.

Look, too, for the yellow sunflower-like blooms that characterize the aptly-named gumweed (*Grindelia integrifolia*). The green bracts surrounding its flowers are covered with a white, very sticky latex or "gum."

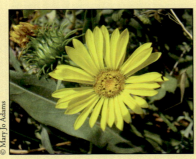

*Gumweed flower*

On protected tideflats, beaches, and salt marshes you may find the distinctive thick, succulent stems of pickleweed (*Salicornia sp.*). One of its common names, glasswort, comes from an historical use of this plant; its salty stems were reduced to ashes to provide sodium carbonate, an ingredient in glassmaking.

# Rainfall in Island County

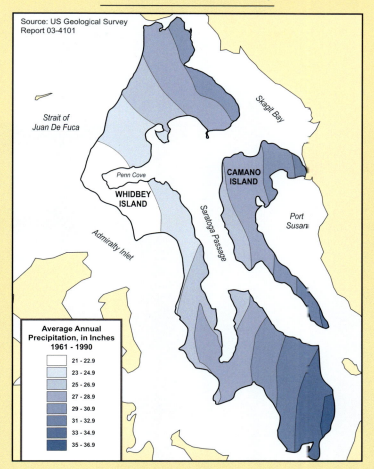

Source: US Geological Survey
Report 03-4101

Strait of
Juan De Fuca

Skagit Bay

Penn Cove

CAMANO
ISLAND

WHIDBEY
ISLAND

Saratoga Passage

Admiralty Inlet

Port
Susan

**Average Annual
Precipitation, in Inches
1961 - 1990**

21 - 22.9
23 - 24.9
25 - 26.9
27 - 28.9
29 - 30.9
31 - 32.9
33 - 34.9
35 - 36.9

We're dry in the middle and wet on the ends. Rainfall varies annually from 21 to 37 inches on different parts of Whidbey and Camano Islands, and microclimates abound. This US Geological Survey rainfall map reveals big differences over a small area. The Olympic Mountains shield the central part of both islands from west-approaching storms, creating a drier area known as a rain shadow. Central Whidbey's fertile agricultural prairies are the driest zone of all, once devoted to dairy production but now trending toward beef production and diversified crops that include small-scale vegetable farms. Farmers capitalize on the drier and warmer winters to over-winter beets and cabbage for seed and to keep soil covered with perennial forage crops and fall-planted grains.

© Sally Slotterback

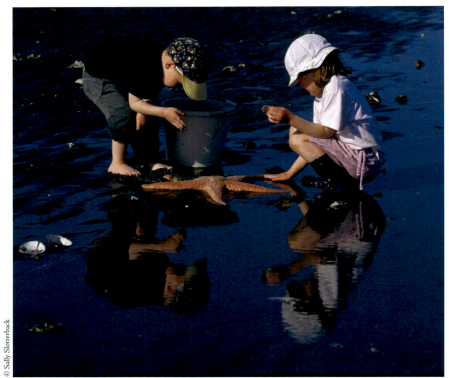

# CHAPTER FOUR

# GUIDE TO INTERTIDAL LIFE

Written and photographed by Mary Jo Adams and Jan Holmes

*For more about intertidal species, see* Sound Water Stewards EZ-ID Guides *at* soundwaterstewards.org/ezidweb/.

## INVERTEBRATES

### Anemones

Early scientists thought anemones were half plant and half animal and it's easy to see why. When the tide covers them and they open, they look much like flowers. They are animals, however, and are in fact carnivores. Anemones have stinging cells in their tentacles, which they use to capture and subdue their prey.

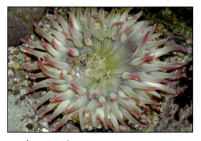

*Aggregating anemone*

The most common species on Island County beaches is the **aggregating anemone** (*Anthopleura elegantissima*). It can grow as a solitary individual or in massive clumps of clones. If in a clump, all others in the clump will be genetically identical. This anemone's green or olive color comes from tiny algae and dinoflagellates that live in its soft tissues.

### Worms, worms, worms

Our intertidal area is littered with hundreds of worm-like creatures that take advantage of both soft sediment and rocky habitats. The most common species fall into three major groups: **marine segmented worms** (polychaetes), **ribbon worms** (nemerteans), and **marine flatworms** (polyclad turbellarians). Polychaete bodies are divided into multiple segments like earthworms. On most polychaetes, each segment is equipped with bristles embedded in flap-like outgrowths. A species' segment structures reflect the lifestyle of the worm. It can be specialized for swimming, burrowing, tube building, and other activities. Polychaete head appendages reflect the worm's diet and food-gathering habits. They range from elaborate feather duster plumes for catching plankton to

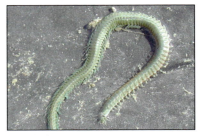
*Polychaete*

protruding jaws and teeth for tearing apart plant and animal material. Many polychaetes are also equipped with elaborate sensory apparatus.

**Nemerteans or ribbon worms** look like pieces of spaghetti or linguini. They have soft, fragile, ciliated bodies that can stretch for yards in some species. The distinctive feature of the group is the remarkable prey-capturing organ, the proboscis. When not in use, it's tucked inside the animal like an inverted finger on a rubber glove. When stimulated by prey, the worm fires its proboscis using hydro-static pressure. The proboscis shoots out, either stabbing the victim with an attached poison stylet or encircling it with sticky prey-quieting secretions. The prey is then engulfed in snake-like fashion. Many nemerteans prefer to eat polychaetes and can ingest animals several times their size.

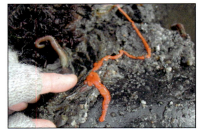
*Ribbon worm*

**Polyclad flatworms** often cling to the underside of rocks or other hard substrates. Their soft, flat, ciliated bodies look like tiny pieces of creeping, flattened chewing gum. The mouth is located in the center of the lower surface

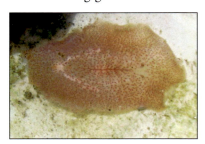
*Flatworm*

and most have conspicuous eyespots on the upper surface. Many flatworm species are known carnivores, feeding on various mollusks, crustaceans, and other marine invertebrates. They evert their pharynx around the prey, then retract it inside to begin digestion. They don't have a complete digestive tract, so undigested material must be passed out through the mouth.

## Snails

Among the more common snails on our beaches are the periwinkles, dogwinkles, and moon snails. All have a raspy tongue-like organ called a radula with which they scrape and drill to procure their food. **Periwinkles** are small, less than an inch long, and live on rocks high up in the intertidal. They crawl along, scraping algae off rocks with their radula. The somewhat larger **dogwinkles**, on the other hand, are predators feeding on mussels and barnacles. You might see clumps of what look like oats on intertidal boulders at certain times of the year. Those are the egg cases of dogwinkle snails.

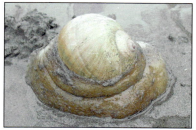

*Moon snail*

Fist-sized **moon snails** live on sandy beaches and spend most of their time plowing along just under the surface of the sand seeking clams. When they find one, they drill through its shell, leaving a circular hole with a countersunk appearance.

After intertidal snails die, their shells are often recycled as homes for hermit crabs.

## Limpets

Limpets look like small, conical hats. As mollusks, they are closely related to snails and chitons and, like them, use a combination of tongue and teeth called a radula. The **plate limpet** (*Tectura scutum*) has a very long radula that measures almost twice the length of its shell. Of course, most of the radula is kept tucked away and the creature uses only a small part of it when feeding.

Limpets are herbivores and make their living scraping thin films of diatoms and algae off intertidal rocks and other surfaces. Limpets are active only when covered by the tide, creeping along the surface of the rock with some species returning to a home spot before the water recedes. They may fall prey to crabs, sea stars, and birds such as the oystercatcher.

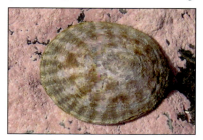

*Plate limpet*

## Chitons

Chitons (pronounced "kitons," which rhymes with "titans") are related to limpets. Instead of one shell, however, they have eight overlapping plates held together by a girdle of tough tissue. This allows them to bend, flex, and conform better to the shape of the rock they are on. Chitons use their radula to scrape algae and other small organisms off rocks. Island County is home to several species, including the **gumboot chiton** (*Cryptochiton stelleri*), the largest species in the world, growing to 13 inches and resembling a large meatloaf. Sometimes

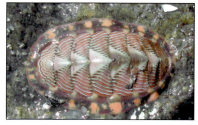

*Lined chiton*

after a storm (especially on west Whidbey Island) gumboot chitons dislodged by the heavy seas can be found tossed up on the beach where they look like half a cantaloupe. Other chiton species found in this area are the colorful **lined chiton** (*Tonicella lineata*), the **black Katy chiton** (*Katharina tunicata*), and the **mossy chiton** (*Mopalia muscosa*). If you find any chiton, please leave it attached to the rock. They cannot reattach very well and probably will not survive if pulled off.

## Clams and mussels

Clams and mussels are mollusks belonging to the bivalve group, their shells being made of two halves joined by a hinge. One or two large muscles keep the shells pulled shut. Both clams and mussels are filter feeders, collecting plankton and other small particles from the water. The most obvious difference between them is that clams generally bury themselves in sand, mud, or other substrate while mussels are right out on the surface, adhering to rocks, pilings, or each other.

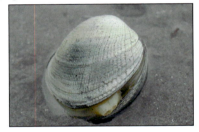
*Littleneck clam*

Look closely at a mussel, and you'll see hair-like strands holding it in place. Called byssal threads, these are secreted as liquid that solidifies into filaments when coming into contact with salt water. Clams have a foot adapted for burrowing. As the clam extends its foot into the sand, the tip of the foot expands and serves as an anchor while the rest of the clam pulls itself down.

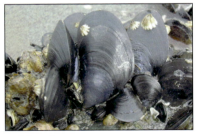
*Mussels*

If you dig clams, please fill the holes when you are finished. Otherwise, piles of sand left on the beach will smother other organisms that live beneath the surface.

## Barnacles

Barnacles are crustaceans, relatives of shrimp, crabs, and beach hoppers. Adult barnacles are permanently attached to some type of substrate, which varies with the species. Some, like the common acorn barnacle, can be found in the intertidal and resemble little stone rosettes attached to rocks. Others reside on the backs of whales and in odd places: one species lives on turtle tongues!

Stalked barnacles such as the goose barnacle live in body chambers attached to a flexible stalk or peduncle, anchored to a hard substrate. Prior to the 1800s some people thought goose barnacles developed into feathered geese!

Unstalked barnacles such as the acorn barnacle have a flat base plate and hard calcareous and overlapping side plates. The base plate is attached to the substrate with barnacle cement, which is stronger than epoxy cement and capable of supporting 7,000 pounds with just one tiny dab. Barnacles knocked off their rock substrates will sometimes leave behind the white base plate giving the rock a snowflaked appearance.

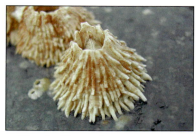

*Thatched barnacle*

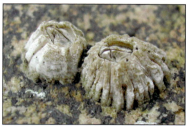

*Acorn barnacle*

Our common **acorn barnacle** (*Balanus glandula*) lives its adult life standing on its head inside its shell. When the barnacle is submerged in seawater, inner plates of the shell open up to expose the cirrus, a fan-like feeding appendage (actually modified legs), which the barnacle uses to comb the water for plankton. Like other crustaceans, the barnacle must periodically molt to increase in size (see box pg. 30). When this happens, the acorn barnacle also enlarges its shell home by dissolving part of the inside of the shell and adding material on the outside.

Barnacles are hermaphrodites: both male and female reproductive organs are present in each individual, but self-fertilization is not common. Barnacles begin life as bristly, one-eyed swimming larvae. When ready for attachment, they metamorphose into a second larval stage to find a suitable attachment spot. Once cemented in place they live as sedentary plankton feeders.

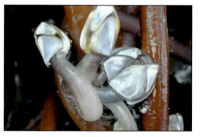

*Pelagic gooseneck barnacle*

Barnacles are harvested commercially for fertilizer and food in some areas. Goose barnacles are popular in Europe as a soup stock base. Barnacles on boat hulls are a serious nuisance organism in maritime communities.

## Shore crabs

Now here's a feisty little guy–the shore crab (genus *Hemigrapsus*). Be ready to get your finger pinched if you pick one up. They have rectangular-shaped carapaces up to two inches wide with three protrusions, called teeth, along the edge behind each eye. Shore crabs are built low-to-the-ground, so they can get under rocks for cover.

*Hemigrapsus nudus*, the **purple shore crab**, usually has purple spots on its claws. Though generally the carapace is purple, you might find one that is olive green or reddish brown and without the purple spots on the claws. Check the walking legs for hair. This species will be hairless. *H. nudus* tends to be found under boulders and in mussel beds on beaches with a fair amount of wave energy.

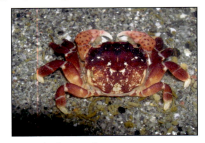

*Purple shore crab*

*Hemigrapsus oregonensis*, the **Oregon** or **green shore crab**, looks similar to *H. nudus* except it has no spots on its claws. Though usually green, carapace color is variable and in juveniles may be white. Look closely for the tiny, bristly hairs on the walking legs that distinguish this species from the purple shore crab. *H. oregonensis* can be found in areas with cobbles and under debris on mudflats. It tends to inhabit somewhat protected waters. *H. nudus* and *H. oregonensis* are sometimes both found on the same beach.

Don't confuse the green shore crab with the invasive **European green crab** (*Carcinus maenas*). The European green crab belongs to a completely different genus and has a fan-shaped rather than rectangular carapace (see box pg. 57).

## Sea stars

Several sea star species live in our waters. They may have five, six, or up to 24 rays (arms) and range from tiny to three feet across. Sea stars move on tube feet controlled by a water vascular system. Look for a spot near the center on their dorsal (top) surface. That is the madreporite, the plate through which seawater enters the vascular system.

One of the most commonly found species, on beaches where the waters are calm, is the **mottled sea star** (*Evasterias troschelii*). It has five slender rays, may reach a foot across, and comes in various colors.

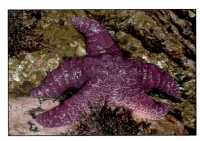

*Purple sea star*

On high-energy beaches such as those on west Whidbey Island, watch for the **purple sea star** (*Pisaster ochraceus*), also called ochre sea star; it can be purple or orange. It may also be a foot across but is much thicker bodied and, in spite of its name, is not always purple. If you find a sea star, please leave it where it is. Pulling it up may damage its tube feet.

# Sea urchins

Sea urchins, which look much like pincushions, are closely related to sea stars and sand dollars. They are herbivores and feed on seaweed. The shell is called a test. Sea urchins have a unique mouthpart called an Aristotle's lantern. Sea urchin spines are attached to the test via ball-and-socket joints that allow them to be used for mobility. The spines are also useful for burrowing and protection.

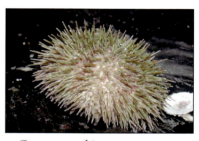
*Green sea urchin*

**Green and purple sea urchins,** found in local waters, belong to the genus *Strongylocentrotus*, which in Greek means "ball of spines," so they are well named.

The **red sea urchin,** *Mesocentrotus franciscanus*, is the largest urchin species on the West Coast and is found from low intertidal to a depth of 400 feet. Some sea urchins live 200 years or longer.

# Sand dollars

Sand dollars are related to sea stars, sea urchins, and sea cucumbers in the phylum Echinodermata. All of these spiny-skinned and strictly marine animals have bodies organized around a water vascular system composed of

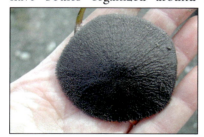
*Sand dollar*

chambers and canals leading to hundreds of tiny tube feet. Sand dollars have an internal shell composed of thousands of little, tightly fitting, plate-like calcareous bones. The flat, ridged sand dollar body plows through sand with its tube feet, collecting small food particles that are channeled into food grooves leading to the mouth. Sand dollars will also orient themselves on edge, letting the plankton-rich water wash over their oral surfaces. If you pick up a living sand dollar, replace it gently on the sand mouth down.

Like urchins, sand dollars grind and chew their food with the remarkable Aristotle's lantern, an inverted cone of five hard pointed teeth. In areas where there is considerable wave action, sand dollars accumulate iron in little internal pockets that serve as weight belts to help stabilize them. In crowded conditions, sand dollars have been observed dislodging other invertebrates and driving them out of sand dollar territory.

Live sand dollars are a rich dark brown or purple with soft felt-like bodies. They are often buried just below the surface in the low intertidal and can easily be overlooked until the beachcomber feels a cookie crunching effect underfoot. Dead specimens are hard and white and often found washed ashore.

# SEAWEEDS

*Seaweeds are large marine algae attached to the sea floor or other substrate by a holdfast. They are non-vascular plants without true roots, stems or leaves. Three common species on our shorelines are bull kelp, rockweed, and sea lettuce.*

## Bull kelp

Just off shore is a forest of seaweed complete with underbrush and canopy layers. One of the tall trees of this forest is the brown seaweed *Nereocystis luetkeana*, or **bull kelp.** Unlike terrestrial trees, bull kelp attains its giant length in just one growing season. It's among the fastest growing photosynthesizing species on the planet, adding about five inches a day and reaching lengths of almost 40 feet (with record specimens up to 118 feet).

Like other seaweeds, bull kelp has no roots and receives no nutrients from the substrate on which it lives. The long blades at the end of its stipe (stem) soak up nutrients directly from seawater. A large, gas-filled bulb at their base keeps

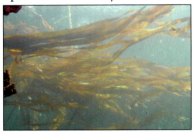
*Bull kelp*

the long fronds afloat. Bull kelp forests provide a safe haven for juvenile fish and a host of invertebrates living on the bottom and in the water column. The kelp is eaten by relatively few animals (among them green sea urchins, which relish it) but provides a rich source of nutrients at the end of its life when it breaks down into small detritus (organic matter and natural debris) particles. Detritus, and the protein-rich microbial colony attached to it, is consumed by a wide variety of marine animals. Humans also consume bull kelp. The blades and stipes are loaded with protein and vitamins and are a favorite ingredient in Asian cooking. Gulls, ducks, and other birds sometimes perch on floating kelp blades, and great blue herons use the kelp beds as platforms from which to fish.

## Rockweed

*Fucus distichus,* or **rockweed,** is widely present along the northern Pacific Ocean. In rocky areas it forms a dense, low-growing canopy that protects numerous invertebrates and other seaweeds from drying out during low tide.

When uncovered by the tide, it's a supple yellow-brown. With increased exposure time, it will darken and become brittle, but rockweed has a high tolerance for exposure extremes. With the exception of small periwinkle snails, few invertebrates eat rockweed because of the polyphenols in its tissues, which inactivate and bind to digestive enzymes of the grazer. On the ends of its branches, mature rockweed has swollen air-filled sacs containing reproductive cells.

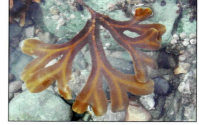

*Rockweed*

Rockweed is used for poultry meal, fertilizer, and garden mulch. It has been consumed by Native Americans for hundreds of years. A favorite time to harvest and consume it is when the swollen tips are hard and dry, like marine popcorn!

## Sea lettuce

This translucent, bright green, leafy seaweed is commonly found during the spring and summer at the mid- to low tide level. Sea lettuce and its many green-bladed relatives can tolerate marine water that has been diluted, so look for it near freshwater sources.

It's a fast-growing, opportunistic species and in some cases can over-grow everything around it, creating blooms. When these blooms occur, seaweeds underneath are deprived of light and the toxic low-oxygen conditions produced when the sea lettuce breaks down can wipe out entire invertebrate and fish communities.

Like many other seaweeds, sea lettuce contains compounds that discourage grazing on it. These are not harmful to humans, however, and sea lettuce is another favorite seaweed in Asian cooking. It's a good source of vitamin C and rich in protein, iron, and iodine.

## Harvesting seaweeds

If you collect sea lettuce or other seaweeds be sure you are far from potential sources of pollution. Wash all seaweed before eating. Over-harvesting or careless cutting of seaweeds can seriously damage a shoreline ecosystem, and whole areas have been denuded of these important algae.

Most state park beaches are closed to seaweed harvest, and elsewhere certain seasons and maximum daily limits apply. A license from Washington Department of Fish and Wildlife is required to collect seaweed. Bull kelp must be cut a minimum of 24 inches above the bulb and short-stemmed kelps at least 12 inches above the anchor point. These rules protect the ability of the seaweeds to reproduce, ensuring their continued presence in the area.

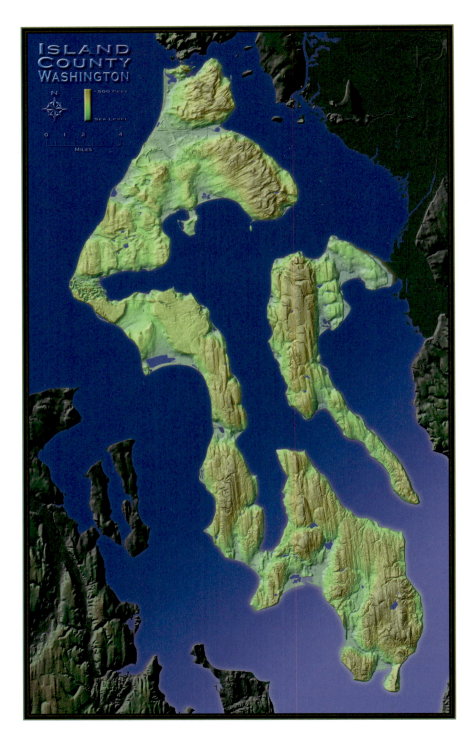

# CHAPTER FIVE

# *Exploring the Edge*

## Explore our glacial and geologic history

This aerial LIDAR (Light Distance and Ranging) map (opposite page) strips away the tree cover and plainly reveals the Ice Age story. Glacially carved north-south bedforms and scars dominate Whidbey and Camano Islands. Keep your eyes open as you travel the islands, and you will catch glimpses of the big picture.

LIDAR measures the terrain accurately to within 30 centimeters vertically (less than a foot) and about 60 centimeters horizontally. GIS (Geographical Information System) technology displays the LIDAR data. Hill shading is added to create a realistic, three-dimensional relief map.

*The LIDAR map of Island County (opposite page) was provided by Island County Public Works, a participant in the Puget Sound LIDAR Consortium (PSLC). PSLC is an informal group of local and federal agencies led by the National Aeronautics and Space Administration (NASA) and the US Geological Survey.*

### Ice meets a barrier at Deception Pass

About 20,000 years ago, during the last of three glacial advances, ice flowed south from the coastal mountains of British Columbia. This "Puget Lobe" of the Vashon Glacier spread into the Puget Sound lowlands and covered Whidbey and Camano Islands to a depth of 3,000 to 5,000 feet. Solid bedrock in the Deception Pass area formed a protective barrier to some degree for the land mass behind it: Whidbey Island.

Once the glacier had blocked the available outflow to the Strait of Juan de Fuca, lakes formed in the Puget Sound basin. Sediment accumulated in these lakes, eventually to be washed away by meltwater from the advancing ice, which gouged the north-south troughs of the Salish Sea.

### Old shorelines still visible

With vast amounts of the world's ocean water tied up in ice sheets, sea level dropped several hundred feet. Offsetting this, the weight of the ice compressed the land below sea level where it remained for thousands of years until the ice melted and the land incrementally rose. The result was the formation of new shorelines, time after time.

These new shorelines are preserved in the geologic record as upland terraces and remain clearly visible on the LIDAR map today in such areas as Livingston Bay on Camano Island, north of Oak Harbor on Whidbey Island, and around Penn Cove near Coupeville.

### Those out-of-place boulders were dropped here

The Puget Lobe of Vashon Glacier carried huge boulders and broke off chunks of rock from nearby mountains such as Mt. Erie, north of Deception Pass on Fidalgo Island. These glacial erratics were later dropped on beaches and in fields and neighborhoods on the two islands as well as elsewhere around the area.

### NE-SW scars are visible north of Oak Harbor

Two exceptions to the predominant north-south orientation of landforms on Whidbey and Camano Islands are an area of NE-SW scarring north of Oak Harbor, and the east-west orientation of Penn Cove. These were formed after the Puget Lobe withdrew and ice from the Cascade mountain glaciers re-advanced down the Skagit River Valley and across north and central Whidbey Island.

### Lake beds and kettles remain

The ice retreated about 13,000 years ago, leaving giant lake beds on central Whidbey. Finer sediments and nutrients flowed into these lakes and settled on the bottom. As the land rose, these lake beds became three fertile prairies that now lie within Ebey's Landing National Historical Reserve (Site 28). The nearby, pock-marked Kettles area consists of many glacial-melt depressions as deep as 200 feet. These were created when large blocks of ice, trapped within the soils at the foot of the receding glacier, melted.

### Mammoths and mastodons roamed here

During interglacial periods, the Puget lowlands provided habitat for mast-odons and mammoths, the bones and tusks of which are found from time to time on the bluffs and beaches of Camano and Whidbey Islands. On Whidbey Island, remnants of these giant mammals have been found near Maxwelton Beach (Site 52) and Scatchet Head. A nearly complete tusk was excavated in the 1960s from a cliff on Camano Island north of Cama Beach (Site 65).

# Watch birds in all their specialized diversity

Birders flock to Island County for its rich diversity of bird species; those noted here are not a complete list. Many loons, grebes, diving ducks, and other water birds are present from fall through early spring. Tropical migrants such as warblers and swallows visit spring through summer while other species reside year round. Highlighted here are some sites particularly good for birding. In the lists of species to look for, the name of a single species is singular (e.g., great blue heron), whereas multiple species or multiple individuals are plural (e.g., scoters, which includes three possible scoter species in the area). A great resource for finding and planning your next bird watching trip is *A Birder's Guide to Washington*, Second Edition, available as a book or at **wabirdguide.org.**

## WHIDBEY ISLAND

A complete island bird list with seasonal occurrences is available on the website of Whidbey Audubon Society, **whidbeyaudubon.org**, where you also can learn about upcoming field trips.

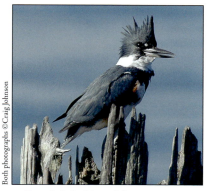

Female belted kingfisher

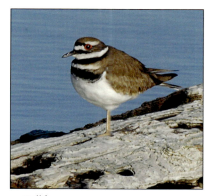

Killdeer

Both photographs ©Craig Johnson

### Deception Pass (Sites 1-4)

Turn west off Hwy 20 into the state park (Site 1) opposite Cornet Bay Rd for rocky sandy shore, tide pools, freshwater wetlands, and rare beach plants. Good for loons, murrelets, black oystercatcher, bald eagle, belted kingfisher, warblers, and other passerines. Turn east onto Cornet Bay Rd (Sites 2-4) for waterfowl in the bay and forest birds in old growth forest at Hoypus Point.

A unique phenomenon occurs in winter, when red-throated loons from throughout the region gather to feed at the maximum outflow from Deception Pass. During the months of December to March, approximately thirty minutes before scheduled high tide at Port Townsend, watch from West Beach and North Beach as hundreds of red-throated loons, as well as Pacific and common loons, grebes, cormorants, mergansers, goldeneyes, pigeon guillemots, and gulls feed in the current flowing out through Deception Pass. The loons gather in long lines offshore, then fly in to feed, drifting out and returning until, sated, they once again gather in long lines offshore before dispersing.

## Dugualla Bay Preserve (Site 7)

Look west from the dike to view birds of freshwater wetland and lakes. East of the dike is a newly-restored tidal estuary and the sheltered water of Dugualla Bay with acres of mudflats at low tide. Look for ducks, shorebirds, great blue heron, osprey, and belted kingfisher. Dugualla Lake is the best place on Whidbey Island to find swans and canvasback in winter.

## Oak Harbor (Sites 11-14)

Oak Harbor beaches and bay offer great blue heron, gulls, cormorants, and abundant waterfowl, including an occasional Eurasian wigeon. In winter, flocks of black turnstone often hang around the marina (Site 11), and picnic nooks along the west end of the marina docks offer close-up looks at grebes and other water birds.

## Joseph Whidbey State Park/Swan Lake/West Beach (Sites 16-17)

In the state park, look for birds of sandy beaches, backshore, cattail marshes, and forests; these birds include savannah sparrow, Virginia rail, marsh wren, warblers, and bald eagle. Swan Lake offers a wide variety of waterfowl including ruddy duck, pintail, shoveler, wigeon, gadwall, bufflehead, coot, and Canada goose as well as shorebirds that include sandpipers, dowitchers, and yellowlegs. Feeding offshore may be loons, grebes, scoters, harlequin duck, and pigeon guillemot.

## Partridge Point (Hastie Lake, Site 18 and Libbey Park, Site 20)

These are prime spots for winter birding. Scan offshore for loons, grebes, pigeon guillemot and other alcids as well as harlequin and long-tailed ducks, scoters, mergansers, and other waterfowl. Black oystercatcher and whimbrel may be seen on the rocky beach below; look for sparrows and wrens in the brush.

## Fort Ebey State Park (Site 21)

Habitats here include second growth forest, thickets, lake, and beach. Birds found include marbled murrelet, mergansers and other water birds, kingfisher, and a great mix of forest species including owls, pileated woodpecker, brown creeper, golden-crowned and ruby-crowned kinglets, flycatchers, and warblers. Enjoy native vegetation and wildflowers along the bluff trails and beach.

## West Penn Cove (Sites 22-23)

On the waters of Penn Cove and in the sheltered lagoons north and west of the cove may be seen abundant water birds such as common and red-throated loons; western and other grebes; cormorants; and ducks, including goldeneyes, scoters, mergansers, and bufflehead. In winter, look on the rocky beaches for shorebirds including black turnstone, surfbird, and sanderling.

## Coupeville Wharf and Captain Coupe Park (Sites 25-26)

Saltwater birds feeding here from fall to spring include loons, grebes, gulls, common and Barrow's goldeneyes, scoters, bufflehead, great blue heron, belted kingfisher, and bald eagle. In summer look for pigeon guillemot and kingfisher nesting in holes in the bluff to the west.

## Ebey's Landing/Bluff Trail/Perego's Lagoon (Site 28)

Trails along bluff and beach offer rare prairie flowers, fields, thickets, forest, backshore lagoon, rocky beach, kelp beds, and offshore waters. You'll see water-oriented birds such as mergansers, scoters, bufflehead, long-tailed duck, cormorants, loons, grebes, killdeer, and yellowlegs. Land birds include red-breasted nuthatch, chickadees, kinglets, warblers, finches, bald eagle, and raven.

## Fort Casey State Park (Sites 29 and 30)

The nutrient-dense waters surrounding the park bring a host of sea birds to this site year-round. From the rocky beach look for water birds including grebes; common, red-throated, and Pacific loons; harlequin duck; rhinoceros auklet; marbled murrelet; pigeon guillemot; and Heerman's and other gulls. Thickets and forest harbor a wealth of woodpeckers, warblers, wrens, sparrows, other passerines, and great horned owl. In summer, migrants like warblers and flycatchers arrive to breed in the forest and along edges.

## Crockett Lake (Site 31)

A top birding location on Whidbey Island, Crockett Lake is a 250-acre brackish marsh and shallow lake formed by Keystone Spit. The lake is a foraging stopover during fall migration for large numbers of shorebirds including dunlin, western and least sandpipers, both dowitchers, black-bellied and semi-palmated plovers, and the occasional godwit, avocet, and other rarities. Waterfowl include scaups, pintail, green-winged teal, shoveler, and hooded merganser. Marshes on the north and east sides are home to American bittern, Virginia rail, and marsh wren. Raptors seen here include peregrine falcon, merlin, northern harrier, bald eagle, and, in winter, short-eared owl and an occasional snowy owl. In summer you can find six swallow species including nesting purple martins. A bird observation platform is located toward the east end of Keystone Spit (pgs. 66-67). Conditions are best for birding when water levels are low, exposing mudflats that are hazardous to walk on. A spotting scope is recommended. Come prepared, take your time, and view birds from a distance. In summer, bird early before heat haze develops.

## South Whidbey State Park (Site 37)

The trail system at this park winds through old growth forest of ancient cedars and firs, home to woodpeckers, Steller's jay, thrushes, western tanager, violet-green swallow, Pacific wren, and small perching birds such as chickadees, kinglets, brown creeper, and red-breasted nuthatch. Osprey nest here. In spring, wander the wide flat trails through the old campground to find breeding warblers and flycatchers.

### Double Bluff Beach (Site 44)

The sandy beach with high bluff offers viewing of gulls, waterfowl, and bald eagle. Great blue heron from a nearby rookery forage on the tideflats and in neighboring Deer Lagoon.

### Deer Lagoon and Sunlight Beach (Sites 45 and 46)

Deer Lagoon is one of the best birding destinations on Whidbey Island. From Deer Lagoon Road, walk the dike to view forest birds. Look for red-winged blackbird, marsh wren, and Virginia rail in the cattails and, on the non-tidal lagoon to the west, many dabbling and diving ducks, coot, and pied-billed grebe. Ospreys and herons perch on old pilings. Since 2016, white pelicans have been coming here in summer to feed and rest. Raptors—including eagles, falcons, and hawks—frequent the area.

The tidal lagoon to the east provides excellent shorebird habitat when mudflats are exposed, with black-bellied plover, dunlin, dowitchers, yellowlegs, small sandpipers, and whimbrel in season. Sunlight Beach accesses provide views into the eastern part of Deer Lagoon, and you can also scope Useless Bay to the south for loons, grebes, scoters, terns, and brant geese.

### Lone Lake (Site 47)

Look for birds of lake, woodlot, and thickets; you may see coot, pied-billed grebe, mergansers, scaups, shoveler, and other waterfowl, as well as Steller's jay, flycatchers, swallows, thrushes, cedar waxwing, yellow and other warblers, red-winged blackbirds, and California quail.

### Langley Seawall Park & Harbor (Sites 49-50)

Birds seen in these saltwater and thicket habitats include cormorants, grebes, loons, mergansers, and other waterfowl as well as bald eagle and small perching birds.

## CAMANO ISLAND & STANWOOD

Learn more about birds in this area from the Camano Wildlife Habitat Project, Friends of Camano Island Parks, and Pilchuck Audubon Society. Birding field trips are offered by Pilchuck Audubon (**pilchuckaudubon.org**) and Skagit Audubon (**skagitaudubon.org**).

### *Camano Island*

### English Boom Historical Preserve (Site 58)

This site is excellent year-round. Look for raptors, loons, scoters, ducks, great blue heron, shorebirds in migration, passerines, and nesting purple martin in summer as well as nesting bald eagle and osprey.

## Utsalady Beach (Site 59)

See birds of deep water such as loons, auklets, scoters, and goldeneyes.

## Maple Grove Park (Site 61)

Saratoga Passage is at its narrowest here and the deep channel is close to shore. Sightings of loons, gulls, harlequin duck, goldeneyes, cormorants, grebes, and alcids such as pigeon guillemot, marbled murrelet, and rhinoceros auklet are possible, as well as rarities like jaegers.

## Livingston Bay (Site 62)

This site is best for ducks at high tide in early morning or late afternoon and for shorebirds when extensive mudflats form at low tide.

## Kristoferson Beaver Marsh

On Can Ku Rd across from the animal shelter, take the short trail to a platform to look out over the beaver marsh for passerines and hooded merganser.

## Iverson Spit Preserve (Site 63)

This site's diverse habitat includes saltwater, mudflats, marsh, and beach, with shrub and cropland nestled against a forested hillside. Iverson Spit is considered a birding hot spot, with over 140 species of birds seen here.

## Four Springs Lake Preserve

This 50-acre preserve, managed by Island County Parks, consists of a mixed coniferous-deciduous forest with a lake and extensive wetlands explored via a one-mile perimeter trail. Bald eagle, pileated woodpecker, and wood duck are common sightings, as well as barred and great horned owls. To get there, go S on East Camano Dr. Turn R on Camano Hill Rd. Turn R on Lewis Lane and follow signs to Four Springs.

## Cama Beach and Camano Island State Parks (Sites 65 and 66)

Hiking trails through diverse habitats—including mixed coniferous-deciduous forest, wetland ponds, and the saltwater of Saratoga Passage—offer bald eagle, harlequin duck, loons, pileated woodpecker, and mixed flocks of chickadees, kinglets, and brown creeper.

## Barnum Point County Park (Site 68)

This park has multiple habitats for good birding with forest, lake, wetlands, and a mile of beach. Trails offer diverse habitat for passerines owls, and woodpeckers. Fall and winter, on the outgoing low tide where the water runs through the tight passage between Triangle Cove and Port Susan Bay, watch for fish-eating ducks and seabirds.

### Stanwood

Stanwood hosts the annual Snow Goose and Birding Festival the last weekend in February with lectures, exhibits, children's activities, and guided bird-watching field trips, including those to locations that are off-limits except during the Festival. From October through March, large flocks of snow geese and tundra and trumpeter swans are frequently seen feeding in fields and heard flying overhead.

## Leque Island Estuary Restoration

Between Camano Island and the City of Stanwood, 2.4 miles of levee were removed from the mouth of the Stillaguamish River to restore 250 acres of diked farmland to tidal marsh habitat. As restoration proceeds, bird varieties will change. Two small boat launches allow access for hand-carry boats, one along Davis Slough and the other along the Stillaguamish River near the Camano Gateway bridge. The latter area also has a tall berm to protect the city of Stanwood from high waves. You'll find a wheelchair-accessible trail that's excellent for viewing wildlife, the restoration in progress, and tidal influences on the river. Directions: watch for signs to two parking areas on the south side of Hwy 532.

## Ovenell City Park

Southeast of the Camano Gateway bridge on the Stanwood side, the City of Stanwood is developing water access to the Stillaguamish River, with a dock for human-powered boats, birding, and dike walks.

## Hamilton Landing

This City of Stanwood park is off of 98th Ave NW at the base of the Hamilton Smokestack and on the shore of the Stillaguamish River. Under development, it's expected to include a trailered boat launch, a hand-carry boat launch, wetlands, and planted buffers. It looks across the river at the wetlands of the Stillaguamish Tribe's *zis a ba* Estuary Restoration Project.

## Stanwood Sewage Lagoon

From Hwy 532 in Stanwood, turn S onto 98th Ave NW. In 225 feet turn L into entrance to Stanwood Waste Water Treatment Plant (limited parking with more at the Hamilton Smokestack). Birders are welcome, but please check in at the office for permission; the gate is open weekdays only. The several ponds, accessed on foot, are excellent for freshwater ducks, gulls, shorebirds in migration, and passerines.

## Thomle and Boe Roads

This winter birding site is located off Marine Dr south of Stanwood on the Stillaguamish delta. The main attractions are snow geese, tundra and trumpeter swans, shorebirds, wintering raptors, and the occasional snowy owl, as well as sparrows in the thickets along Thomle Rd.

# View whales from shore in spring and fall

The top whale-watching seasons in Island County are spring and fall, though sightings are possible year-round. Gray whales and orcas visit the Whidbey and Camano shorelines every year and when present may be seen from almost any place with a good view of the water.

A small group of seasonally resident gray whales visit our waters from March through early June, especially in Saratoga Passage where they feed in areas of sandy or muddy shallows where ghost shrimp reside (see box pgs. 91-92). **On Whidbey Island**, the best places to look for gray whales are in Penn Cove (Sites 19, 23-27); Hidden Beach (Site 34); Worm Road (Site 35); in the sandy shallows directly off the Langley waterfront and marina (Sites 49, 50); and at Possession Point on the southern tip of the island (Sites 56, 57). **On Camano Island**, gray whales can be seen from viewpoints overlooking Saratoga Passage and Port Susan waters (Sites 65, 66, 68) Whale watching boats indicate their presence, or on quiet evenings you may hear their blows after dark.

Resident orcas (see box p. 79) are seen off west Whidbey Island, in Saratoga Passage, and in Possession Sound, usually October through January. Transient orcas travel regularly through Island County waters and can show up at any time, peaking in April and August. The best places to view orcas **on Whidbey Island** are West Beach Vista (Site 17); Libbey Beach (Site 20); Fort Ebey (Site 21); Ebey's Landing bluff (Site 28); Fort Casey (Site 29); Lagoon Point (Sites 36A, 36B); Bush Point (Sites 38, 39); Clinton pier or ferry dock (Site 54); Glendale (Site 55); and Possession Point (Sites 56, 57). **On Camano Island**, the west side occasionally offers views of orcas (Sites 59, 61, 65, 66).

On the Facebook page and website **orcanetwork.org**, Orca Network posts recent sightings, and the Facebook page Camano Whale Watchers posts updates on whales seen from Camano Island. Please report whale sightings to 1-866-ORCANET or info@orcanetwork.org. Orca Network provides data collected through their Whale Sightings Network to NOAA Fisheries and other research organizations. You may join the sightings e-mail list at **orcanetwork.org**. To get an idea of the soundscape whales live in, listen to the Bush Point hydrophones at **orcasound.net.**

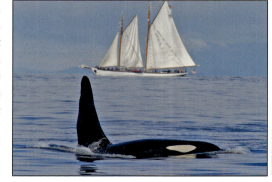

© David Ellifrit

# Go kayaking for a quiet, close view of nature

Kayaking is a tranquil way to experience the beauty and diversity of the islands' special places. It brings us quietly close to nature and affords time to see, hear, and smell, and take pictures with minimal disturbance of the setting.

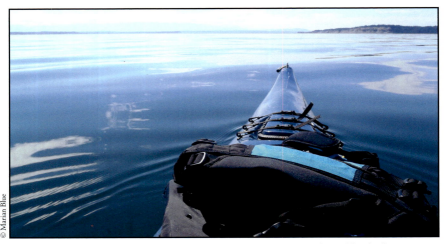

© Marian Blue

*Kayaking in quiet waters off Maxwelton Beach, looking toward Double Bluff*

### *Prepare carefully for a safe trip*

The rapidly changeable weather, currents, tides, and winds around the islands require great respect, careful preparation, and wise judgment.

- Know your limits. Avoid kayaking alone unless you're very experienced.
- Check tides, currents, and wind forecasts before setting out. Tides cause currents, but currents do not necessarily follow tides, so consult both a tide table and a current table. Wind is a particular concern around Whidbey Island, and it generally picks up in the afternoons, sometimes very quickly.
- Puget Sound's numbingly cold water temperatures year-round can quickly disable people in the water, allowing little time for rescue. Be trained in safety procedures and have practiced self-rescue and re-entry. Learn the buddy-assisted wet exit rescue technique; local lakes on Whidbey Island—such as Deer and Goss Lakes—are ideal practice areas. Voluntary organizations such as Whidbey Island Sea Kayakers (WISK) offer training sessions, as does Whidbey Island Sea Kayaking Company.
- Dress with the expectation that you will get wet. Wear a wetsuit or a drysuit in addition to layered and windproof clothing, and use a spray skirt. Wet clothing can drain heat from your body, causing hypothermia, even without immersion. Wear a personal flotation device at all times.

- Carry the "10 essentials of kayaking," including first aid supplies; extra food, water, and clothing; bilge pump and paddle float; a water to shore signaling/radio device (VHS recommended); a hat; and sunscreen. Keep all supplies in water-tight containers. You may want to include binoculars and a camera.
- Share your trip plan with a friend or neighbor, and let them know when you've returned. It's a good idea to post your trip plan on the dashboard of your car.

### Getting started

If you're a first-timer, try a guided tour. Learn about kayaking through books, training videos, or websites, which can also provide purchasing advice for kayaks, paddles, and the related equipment you will need

### Give marine mammals and birds their space

The Marine Mammal Protection Act requires all craft to stay at least 100 yards from whales (the length of a football field), 200 yards away from orcas and designated bird sanctuaries in Washington State waters, and 50 feet from dolphins, porpoises, seals, and sea lions. Seals need time out of water to keep warm. Give wide berth to what appear to be abandoned harbor seal pups. Their mothers will return to retrieve them. Binoculars are the best way to get a closer look.

*The following are descriptions of some kayak routes around Island County. Site numbers refer to site descriptions in Chapter 3.*

## WHIDBEY ISLAND

The direction and velocity of both wind and current matter a great deal when kayaking Whidbey Island's shoreline, as does knowledge of how tide height affects launching sites. Have a car at both your starting and ending points, and you won't have to struggle against strong winds or currents back to your starting point. Perhaps start your day at a launch point best used only at high tide and end at one where the tide level is not a serious issue—or vice versa.

These routes were compiled by volunteers who kayaked all of Whidbey Island's 150+ miles of shoreline except for the challenging and dangerous waters of Deception Pass. Updated information was provided by Whidbey Island Sea Kayakers (WISK). These sites are a sampling of all the public access points needed to circumnavigate Whidbey Island; any of them can be used for round trips. For more extensive information, search online for "Island Beach Access WISK," and click on the region where you would like to kayak.

Deception Pass and nearby waters should not be attempted by any but the most qualified and experienced kayakers, preferably with an experienced guide and after careful preparation. Anacortes-based Hole in the Wall Paddling Club provides a Kayaking Skill Level Matrix that assigns a number to each site based on geography, conditions, and hydraulics. It should be reviewed before going on any paddle. Always be honest with yourself about your current skill level and check up-to-date forecasts. For information on the skill level matrix and more, visit **holeinthewallpaddlingclub.org.**

## Ala Spit (Site 5), north end, east side

Pack a picnic lunch and enjoy a full day paddling to either Hope Island, a Washington State Park Natural Area Preserve, or Skagit Island. After crossing the channel to Hope Island, paddle the north side of the island and go ashore at the bay landing site to enjoy your picnic and explore designated trails. Skagit Island, slightly to the north, is another gem. It also has a wonderful lunch spot, a trail circumnavigating the island, and a couple of overnight campsites (but no potable water).

When crossing, note that the current is swift on the west shoreline, so it's very important to pay attention to the tides. Even though it's a few miles away, Ala Spit is affected by the massive tidal flow through Deception Pass. As the gap between the easterly top of Ala Spit and Hope Island narrows, the current flow intensifies. Avoid launching or landing at low tides at Ala Spit, as you will find yourself transporting your kayak a considerable distance to and from the parking lot.

Another way to enjoy this area is to launch at the Deception Pass State Park dock in Cornet Bay (Site 3) on an incoming tide (flood tide), and then end your day at Ala Spit (leave a car in both places). Cornet Bay is a well-established site with many amenities, including potable water and restrooms, making this an ideal place to begin a kayaking session. Watch for swift currents and always exercise caution paddling in Deception Pass waters. First paddle east, then south around Hoypus Point, a shoreline where you'll probably see sandpipers and other shorebirds. From Hoypus Point, paddle out to catch a flood current over to Skagit Island, and then paddle down to and around Hope Island. Enjoy your picnic lunch on either island, where birding is excellent. End your adventure by paddling at high slack tide across the channel from Hope Island to Ala Spit, landing on the sandy, south-facing side of the spit. Keep an eye out for seasonal changes in driftwood at Ala Spit, which could make exiting the site a challenge.

Alternatively, you could paddle from Ala Spit to Dugualla Bay (Site 7). It's further south and a somewhat easier paddle, but be sure to exit at high tide because the bay turns into a mud flat at low tide.

## Penn Cove (Sites 19, 22, 26), north-central island, east side

This is a delightful place, offering beautiful views of historic Coupeville from the water. It's easy to launch at any of the three sites. Paddle around

Coupeville Wharf and observe the numerous sand dollars west of the wharf, the sea stars attracted to the mussels on the pilings, and the moon and egg yolk jellyfish floating in the water. The mussel rafts one-mile west are fascinating when mussels are being harvested, cleaned, and packed; harbor seals and their pups often lounge on these rafts. Please respect this private property.

Another half-mile further is the historic Captain Whidbey Inn, a possible lunch stop. You may glimpse John Colby Stone's classic 52-foot ketch, Cutty Sark. Penn Cove is designated as an Important Bird Area by Audubon Washington. You'll see ducks, loons, and grebes on the water; shorebirds and great blue heron along the beaches and rocky shores as well as in Grasser's Lagoon; and raptors sailing overhead.

## Monroe Landing (Site 19)

Launch here and paddle west along the north shore towards Grasser's Lagoon (Site 22). This trip offers views of the Cascade and Olympic Mountain ranges, as well as Coupeville and the mussel farm. The shoreline at the west end of Penn Cove is often muddy at low tide. Watch for wind if crossing south to Coupeville.

## Captain Coupe Park (Site 26)

A few blocks east of Coupeville, this park with a boat ramp offers an ideal launch site. Avoid this ramp at low tides because it's surrounded by mud.

Don't plan to launch from the Coupeville waterfront shoreline as it is inhospitable; however, it is possible to rent a kayak at the end of the wharf.

Wherever you launch, make sure to check your tide tables. Landing at one of these sites during low tide could leave you stranded in mud or with a very long walk to your vehicle.

## Long Point (Site 27)

Located at the eastern tip of Penn Cove, this site offers views of Mount Baker and Oak Harbor, but wind may be a problem.

## Ebey's Landing (Site 28) central island, west side

Plan to launch from this site on a calm day or before the surf comes up, unless you are agile enough to jump into your kayak between waves while standing in water up to your knees. Also, the walk to the water's edge will be shorter and easier if you launch at high tide. If you're planning to kayak between Ebey's Landing and Fort Ebey State Park (Site 21), wind and current direction and velocity make a difference.

This is a pleasant paddle with lovely views of Ebey's Bluff from the water. A nice interlude from paddling is to go ashore briefly at Perego's Lagoon to view both the lagoon and wildlife around it. The beach at Fort Ebey State Park is a reasonably easy place to either launch or end your excursion. However, the walk back to the parking lot is uphill and a little long. If you find it easier to carry your kayak downhill than uphill, and the wind and currents allow, launch at Fort Ebey State Park and haul out at Ebey's landing.

Alternatively, you could launch or land at Keystone Jetty (Site 30), making a lovely 4-mile paddle, in one direction, from Ebey's Landing. You will need to be wary of the wake caused by ferries and strange currents in the area, both of which can be managed with diligence and planning. For more information on kayaking at Keystone Jetty, see below. Driftwood Park (Site 32) is another great spot to launch and paddle to Ebey's Landing.

**Keystone Jetty (Site 30), west side**

Launch at the boat ramp in the harbor. When tides are extreme, the current can be strong at the end of the jetty. The waters along the east side of the jetty and extending to the wooden pier are a marine conservation area, popular with divers. The marine life is extraordinary; divers report more than 50 fish species and 40 invertebrate species including the giant Pacific octopus. It's fun to explore around the abandoned wooden pier where marine life is abundant on the pilings and birds congregate on top. Pigeon guillemots nest in crevices of the old pier in summer; all three species of cormorants perch on top. For a longer paddle, launch at Ebey's Landing (Site 28) and head south to the harbor. Be sure to watch for the ferry and be very careful of the tricky shoals just to the west of the harbor entrance. Another alternative, especially attractive if you have two cars, is to continue south to Ledgewood Beach (Site 33).

**Ledgewood Beach (Site 33), west side**

This launch site requires carrying the boat down a gravel ramp and over rocks to the beach, but it's an enjoyable place to kayak if you have time for only a short excursion. Paddle north around some big rocks for good looks at intertidal invertebrates and a nice variety of brown algae nearby. The lion's mane jellyfish may be seen in this area. Other than a trip to Keystone Jetty, you could make a slightly longer trip to Lagoon Point South (Site 36B), past a bird sanctuary at the midway point (Lake Hancock). This is a Navy restricted area, so please respect the no trespassing signs. South of the Ledgewood Beach access, you can see what remains of the 2013 Ledgewood landslide.

**Bush Point Boat Launch (Site 38), west side**

Launch from this site at a minus outgoing tide (-2 or below) on a day when there is virtually no wind and the water is clear. Paddle north close enough to the shore to keep no more than 3-6 feet of water under your kayak. About ¾ mile from your launch point, and extending another ¾ mile north, are incredible displays of brown algae. Algae species include *Alaria marginata*, *Costaria costata*, *Mazzaella splendens*, *Saccharina latissima*, and *Sargassum muticum*. Amongst the blades you may see jellyfish, sea cucumbers, crabs, and countless other species as well as rhinoceros auklets and pigeon guillemots on the water. It's a good idea to both begin and end this excursion at Bush Point as the currents are often wildly confusing and difficult to deal with at Lagoon Point, 3 miles north of Bush Point. Also, there can be very strong currents at the western tip of Bush Point, so use extreme caution. This launch site becomes crowded during fishing season, with shore- and boat-based fishermen casting their lines in all directions. Salmon fishing from a kayak is quite a thrill, and Bush Point is an ideal place to try it—but you won't be alone.

## Holmes Harbor (Sites 41, 35), south island, east side

Put in at Freeland County Park (Site 41) and paddle out around Baby Island at the mouth of Holmes Harbor. Be aware that this is a long paddle, and prevailing afternoon winds can make it difficult, but you may get a push on the return by a breeze from the north. Know your tides, as dangerous and unwalkable mudflats abound. Baby Island is a haul-out for harbor seals and their pups; they are very curious and may swim near your kayak, popping up for a look.

If Baby Island is your kayaking destination, Wonn Road (Site 35) makes for a pleasant and much shorter paddle. You may use the private drive to unload your kayak but must park your car at Greenbank Farm. Paddling to Baby Island requires crossing the mouth of Holmes Harbor, an open-water crossing of about 1.5 miles, best done in the morning or early afternoon.

## Mutiny Bay (Site 42, 43), west side

Robinson Beach (Site 42) and Limpet Lane (Site 43) offer access to Mutiny Bay, a wide, relatively protected site with grand homes and excellent sunsets. The seabird life is rich, including scoters and pigeon guillemots. In summer, pigeon guillemots nest in burrows in the bluffs south of Mutiny Bay. Bald eagles frequent the trees on the bluff. In season, Mutiny Bay can have great conditions for kayak fishing.

## Useless Bay (Site 46), west side

This launch site in the Sunlight Beach area (Site 46) offers access to Useless Bay through the channel to Deer Lagoon, a wonderful site for bird watching. Useless Bay is very shallow and protected from north winds. Avoid this bay in the event of strong south winds, and at low tide the bay turns into extensive mudflats. Use caution kayaking around to Deer Lagoon. It is extremely shallow, and it's easy to be trapped in the mudflats at low tide.

## South Whidbey Harbor at Langley (Site 50), east side

You can launch and return to this site at a low or high tide. Depending on the wind velocity and direction, you can have a nice paddle either north or south. If you go south, you may see shorebirds, loons, Bonaparte's gulls, western grebes, and bald eagles around Sandy Point. Along the way, enjoy the lovely shoreline with overhanging trees. You'll eventually reach Clinton Beach Park (Site 54) next to the ferry dock. In spring, paddle north a few miles when the tide is out, and you may spot gray whale feeding pits in the exposed mud and sand along the shoreline; you may even see a gray whale! Be careful just offshore from the town of Langley at low tide. If you get hung up in the mud, you will not be able to step out and re-launch in deeper water.

### Clinton Beach Park (Site 54), east side

This park, adjacent to the ferry, is an excellent launch and haul out location. Parking space is limited, so plan ahead.

### Dave Mackie Waterfront Park (Site 52), west side

Time your launches and returns to this site close to a high tide because at low tide it's a long walk from the water's edge to the parking lot. Determine the direction and velocity of wind and current, and decide if you want to paddle north or south. For a short excursion, paddle north through shallow waters to view what appears to be a nursery for sand dollars. If a breeze picks up, hug the shore.

### Possession Beach Waterfront Park (Site 57), southeast side

This day-use park is ideal for kayakers. It offers an improved launch for all kinds of watercraft, ample parking, fresh water, and, often, protection from the wind. Paddling to the southern tip of the island provides views of the Seattle skyline, as well as the Olympics and Cascades. Waterfowl are abundant, bald eagles frequent the area, and harbor seals often rest themselves on the large rocks jutting out from shore. Adventurous paddlers can continue westward around the tip of Whidbey to the entrance to Cultus Bay. Here you are almost halfway to Maxwelton Beach if you want to extend your trip even farther. Be aware that prevailing winds and currents shift as you pass from the east to the west along the southern tip of the island; turn around if troublesome. Winds are usually manageable, making this an ideal outing.

## BOWMAN BAY AND ROSARIO HEAD, FIDALGO ISLAND

Just north of Deception Pass in Skagit County is another great kayaking opportunity not to be overlooked.

Bowman Bay and Rosario are part of Deception Pass State Park on Fidalgo Island. Bowman Bay is easily reached from Hwy 20. About 0.5 mile N of Deception Pass, turn W on Rosario Rd and take the first L. This is a good place to launch at any tide and is superb for protected paddling. Rosario Park is farther down Rosario Rd, but you will have a long carry to launch there. Bowman Bay is a better launch site and in good conditions is a relatively safe paddle if you don't venture south of the Bowman Bay entrance, which will bring you too close to Deception Pass.

Head west out of the bay and turn north to take in the view of Rosario Head, exploring the exposed rocks along the way. At low tide, you can meet the sea creatures that other park visitors don't see. Unlike the glacial substrates that comprise most of Island County's bluffs and beaches, this area is exposed bedrock. The steep rocks and sheer cliffs reveal a rich diversity of intertidal life, including chitons, predatory dogwinkle snails, the bread-crumb sponge, large colorful anemones of the genus *Urticina*, and handsome purple and orange sea stars, *Pisaster ochraceus*. A large bed of bull kelp rings Rosario Head and a variety of other seaweeds can be seen growing on the rocks. Turn in toward Rosario beach, and if you're lucky, you may get a good look at the oystercatchers—large black shorebirds with bright red bills and feet—that nest on the small islands northwest of Rosario Head. Continue north about ¼ mile to a small cave. Best at low tide, nose your kayak in to see white plumose anemones, *Metridium* sp., adorning the walls.

## CAMANO ISLAND

Around Camano Island, it's the tide and winds, more than currents, that determine where and when to kayak. It's particularly important to stay aware of tide levels. These are suggestions for kayak excursions from public access points, and in most cases the next nearest launch and landing site is identified for those with a shuttle car.

Camano Island's four paved boat ramps receive heavy traffic when crabbing season is open, especially on weekends. Always exercise caution when entering water with motorized boats and avoid their wake.

The Shoreline Photo Viewer from the Department of Ecology is an excellent online resource to plan and visualize your next trip: **fortress.wa.gov**, search "Shoreline Photo Viewer."

### English Boom Preserve (Site 58)

Launching and landing a kayak here is advisable only at higher tides as there are extensive tidal flats. At higher tides, this is the closest launch and landing site for the mouth of the West Pass of the Stillaguamish River. (See also Site 59.)

### Utsalady Boat Ramp (Site 59)

Usable at all tide levels, this boat ramp is very heavily used by motorized vessels and commercial crab boats, so parking can be very tight. Paddling to the east and then north around the bluffs of Arrowhead Point brings the kayaker into Skagit Bay. Time the tides carefully, and you can paddle about 4 miles to English Boom Park, on into the mouth of the Stillaguamish River, and back to Arrowhead Point. The farther east you paddle from Arrowhead Point, the more tide flats you encounter, so it's important to check your tides. At mid to low tides, you may see seals hauled out on sand islands in the middle of Skagit Bay. Paddling 3.5 miles to the west and south around Utsalady Point brings you to Maple Grove County Park (Site 61). Currents around Utsalady Point can be challenging, so always plan ahead and be prepared.

## Maple Grove County Park (Site 61)

The paved boat ramp here is good for launching at low tide, and there is ample parking except during crabbing season weekends. Paddling east and north brings you to an intertidal area of clay-like substrate with shallow pools containing hundreds of anemones. This is the closest thing to tide pools on Camano Island.

Be aware of unpredictable currents as you continue around rocky Utsalady Point, past shoreside homes, and to the Utsalady Boat Ramp (Site 59). Leaving the boat launch, paddle west then south, toward the Madrona neighborhood of Camano. This shoreline offers views of sloughing bluffs and several spots for beaching your boat to go ashore, stretch your legs, or go swimming. Watch for eagles, kingfishers, herons, seals, bull kelp, and boaters (especially during crabbing season).

## Livingston Bay (Site 62)

Fox Trot Way provides kayak launching only at higher tides; otherwise, it would be necessary to carry over extensive mud flats and much driftwood. The main attraction is bird watching as the bay provides habitat for many water birds. A determined paddler could launch and land here to paddle 2-3 miles to Iverson Spit (Site 63), which also has extensive tide flats and a considerable carry over driftwood.

## Iverson Spit Preserve (Site 63)

See Livingston Bay above. Paddle south from Iverson Spit to pass several communities of shoreside homes and travel around the bluffs of Barnum Point (Site 68). Explore Triangle Cove or continue to Cavalero Park (Site 64) in about 3 miles from Iverson Spit.

## Cavalero Park (Site 64)

Cavalero Park has a boat ramp, so it's possible to launch a kayak at most tides in spite of the tide flats. The geography at this launch site provides some protection from westerly winds. As you paddle north and east along Driftwood Shores spit, the reason for the name is evident. Most of the spit is private property with tightly packed houses. At the east end of the spit is the entrance to Triangle Cove where it's possible to enter at most tides, but the best paddling is from mid to high tides. This is a favorite area to observe various birds in season. Eagles and herons are commonly seen fishing the channels, and various ducks and seabirds feed on the tide flats. Invasive *Spartina* grass has essentially been eradicated but monitoring continues. There is a small oyster-growing effort on private tidelands in Triangle Cove.

Paddlers should be aware of possible currents crossing the entrance to Triangle Cove. At high tidal exchanges, experienced kayakers can play in some Class 1 currents. After crossing the entrance to Triangle Cove, the paddler comes to Barnum Point County Park (Site 68), which has no direct access to launch a kayak, but once on the water, there are two access points from the beach to the upland trails. The western upland trail access is located directly after crossing the channel to Triangle Cove. The second upland trail access is a mile farther east. In between, the mile of beach offers kayakers a chance to stretch their legs and explore. There are no facilities on the beach; please be respectful. Off the western edge of Barnum Point, the paddler will note several glacial erratic boulders off the beach (see box pg. 89). The distance to the current feeder bluff (see box pg. 85) gives a hint of how much the bluff has eroded since glacial times. An energetic paddler could continue on to Iverson Spit (Site 63).

Paddling south from Cavalero Park brings you along bluffs where the houses sit high above, and pigeon guillemots have burrowed into the sandy bluff. After a short while, you're paddling by the shoreline homes of the Country Club development. Beach access at Country Club is limited to residents of the development.

## Cama Beach State Park (Site 65)

There is no public kayak launch/retrieval available at the park. Seasonally, you can rent a kayak or rowboat. To kayak here, launch at Camano Island State Park (Site 66).

## Camano Island State Park (Site 66)

You can launch a kayak at any tide level from this boat launch located in an area of fairly steep gravel beaches. Paddle to the north several miles for an opportunity to visit Cama Beach State Park (Site 65) with its 1930s era cabins, boathouse, and store. You can land on the shoreline to enjoy the historic area and park trails; the Cama Beach store is a popular source for ice cream bars. This stretch of Saratoga Passage is subject to afternoon winds, and there is considerable boat traffic close to shore, so keep an eye out for boat wakes.

Paddle to the south, then east around Point Lowell, to one of the few areas on Camano with bull kelp beds (see box pgs. 49-50). Continue east along the shore to Elger Bay. In spring, look for eagles and gray whales. Elger Bay has tide flats, but at mid to high tide, it's possible to explore up into the blind channels of the estuary behind the Elger Bay spit. Exploring the channels is recommended for fairly short kayaks only because turn-around opportunities are limited.

To avoid powerboat traffic at the boat launch, and for more protection from west and north winds, park at the very south end of the parking lot and launch from there.

### Tillicum Beach (Site 67)

At this small neighborhood park with limited parking, it's sometimes necessary to carry over driftwood. When the tide is out, there's a nice gravel beach. Mud flats are a problem only at the very lowest tides, so plan to return or launch at this site at higher tides. Paddle north, approximately 6 miles, along residential areas on the beach and the bluff to Cavalero County Park (Site 64). Paddle south, passing shoreline residential areas and a beach area with little noticeable human intrusion, until you round the south tip at Camano Head. Camano Head shows evidence of a large landslide resulting from a local tsunami in the early 1800s. As you paddle around Camano Head, you're again near residential areas. Please respect private property and do not haul out without permission from landowners.

## Kayak Camps

The Washington Water Trails Association lists eight kayak camps in Island County or nearby waters. These campsites are intended only for those arriving by water in a non-motorized beachable boat. They are among more than 50 such camps located along the Cascadia Marine Trail, a saltwater trail spanning more than 140 miles from the Canadian border to southernmost Puget Sound near Olympia. This inland sea trail is a National Recreation Trail, one of only 16 National Millennium Trails designated by the White House. Campsites are suitable for day use or multi-day trips and may be reached from many public and private launch sites or shoreline trailheads. More information and a more exhaustive list of camp sites are available online from the Washington Water Trails Association, **wwta.org**. Kayak camps are located at:

- Deception Pass State Park - Bowman Bay (Fidalgo Island)
- Hope Island Marine State Park
- Skagit Island State Park
- Ala Spit County Park (Site 5)
- Joseph Whidbey State Park (Site 16)
- Fort Ebey State Park (Site 21)
- Possession Point State Park (Site 56)
- Camano Island State Park (Site 66)

# Fish for dinner or just for peace

Many beaches on the western shore of Whidbey Island offer exceptional shore fishing (see box pgs. 75-76). Fishing offers opportunities to do some clear thinking, learn about nature, make a new friend, and teach a child good habits.

### Courtesy and etiquette keep anglers welcome

The most welcome anglers on the beach are those who keep the big picture in mind. They politely ask permission, offer a hand to others, give space to their neighbor, and pick up debris. They know that a few minutes of courtesy make all the difference in keeping recreational opportunities open. They take only the fish they will consume, use proper catch-and-release methods, and pick up stray monofilament line and hooks to leave the beach cleaner and safer for wildlife and humans who will follow. They promote ethical behavior and public awareness of conservation issues. They not only catch fish, but they also make it their business to be advocates for the fish and for healthy marine habitats.

To find when and where to fish for salmon, how to identify our five salmon species, current regulations, and other resources, go to wdfw.wa.gov, and search "recreational salmon fishing."

## Some Island County fishing beaches

| Site | Name | Site | Name |
|------|------|------|------|
| 1 | Deception Pass State Park (salt and fresh water) | 37 | South Whidbey State Park |
| | | 38 | Bush Point Boat Launch |
| 2 | Cornet Bay County Dock | 39 | Bush Point - Sandpiper Road |
| 3 | Cornet Bay Boat Launch Pier | 43 | Mutiny Bay Shores |
| 5 | Ala Spit County Park | 47 | Lone Lake (fresh water) |
| 11 | Oak Harbor City Marina | 48 | Goss Lake (fresh water) |
| 12 | Pioneer Way East | 50 | S. Whidbey Harbor Fishing Pier |
| 13 | Flintstone Park | 53 | Deer Lake (fresh water) |
| 21 | Fort Ebey State Park | 54 | Clinton Beach Pier |
| 22 | Grasser's Lagoon | 55 | Glendale Beach Preserve |
| 28 | Ebey's Landing | 56 | Possession Point State Park |
| 29 | Fort Casey State Park | 57 | Possession Beach Waterfront Park |
| 31 | Keystone Spit | 63 | Iverson Spit Preserve |
| 32 | Driftwood Beach Park | 65 | Cama Beach State Park |
| 36A | Lagoon Point North | 66 | Camano Island State Park |
| 36B | Lagoon Point South | 68 | Barnum Point County Park |

# Go clamming for buried treasure

Clamming is like going after treasure: you might get lucky, it's good family fun, and can be great eating. Help keep clamming available by knowing what you're doing, so you won't unintentionally harm clams and other marine life. Respect private property by staying within public beach boundaries. Follow these guidelines:

**1. Stay alive.** Make absolutely certain the beach where you plan to dig is not closed by the Department of Health (DOH). To know the status of a beach for both biotoxins and pollution, go to **doh.wa.gov** and **wdfw.wa.gov** and search "shellfish safety"; additionally, call the state Shellfish Safety Hotline, 1-800-562-5632. Certain toxins sometimes present in shellfish are not killed by cooking or freezing and can be deadly. Conditions can change quickly, so always check the WA shellfish safety sites and call the Hotline the same day you plan to dig.

**2. Avoid a ticket** and help conserve our shellfish resource. Before you dig on public beaches, you are required by law to have a state Shellfish/Seaweed or Combo License (available at hardware stores, other outlets, and online). To ensure clams for future generations, the state tracks recreational harvests and limits harvest seasons when necessary, so be aware of beach-specific harvest seasons. Know current daily bag limits, minimum size restrictions, oyster shucking requirements, year-round pollution closures, and other rules (available online or where you buy your license). Check the Shellfish Safety Hotline and consult a tide chart for the beach you plan to visit. You may also check the WDFW Shellfish Rule Change Hotline, 1-866-880-5431. An absence of emergency rules means permanent rules are in effect.

**3. Refill all the holes you dig.** This is the law, and it's the right thing to do. Clams, mussels, oysters, and other marine life can suffocate under piles of sand or rocks left behind while digging holes. Most of these animals are unable to relocate themselves. Clams can be killed by warmer water that collects in unfilled holes and is heated by the sun before the tide comes in. Many clams are lost to currents and gulls from unfilled holes. Unfilled holes

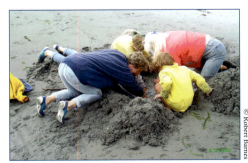

*Digging for geoduck*

are a hazard, especially for small children and mobility-impaired individuals walking on an uneven beach. Push any undersized clams into the refilled hole.

**4. Replace clams properly.** Most clams can't right themselves, nor dig upwards, so if you put them back wrong, they will die. As you refill the hole, do your best to replace undersized or excess clams exactly as you found them. Replace each clam at its proper depth, one to two times as deep as the length of its shell. Bury small clams too deep, and they will suffocate; bury big clams too shallow and they can be picked off by gulls.

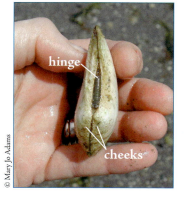

© Mary Jo Adams

Place the clam with its siphon (neck) up and its foot down, no deeper than the length of its neck; the siphon/neck must reach the surface to extract food and oxygen from the water.

To tell which way is up when the shell is closed, note the bulge just below the hinge. The growth rings radiate from this bulge. The clam's neck protrudes above the hinge. Always replace a clam vertically, with the bulges (cheeks) down, below the hinge.

*Rules to remember for replacing clams:*

1. *Place vertically, with cheeks below the hinge.*
2. *Place no deeper than twice the length of its shell.*

**5. Know your clam types, limits, and habitats.** Knowing about the clam you're after can save a lot of trouble and damage to the resource. Can you recognize the size and shape of the holes it leaves? How deep does it go? Which shovel or tool works best? Which direction will it dig, so you won't dig into it and break it in half?

Know the current regulations and current limits before you dig. Sign up for a Digging 4 Dinner class given on Whidbey by Sound Water Steward volunteers (see **soundwaterstewards.org**).

**6. Carry a bucket for clams and safety.** Walking on saturated lower beaches and tide flats can quickly turn scary and even dangerous. At times it may become impossible to walk on tidal mud without being sucked in. A bucket's wide base can be a safety tool to help you gain leverage to pull a foot out of the mud. If you try to turn around you'll get sucked in deeper, so back up and retrace your steps.

**7. Handle and store your catch safely.** Review state and county health departments' websites and follow their recommendations. These include:

- Rinse your catch in salt water, not fresh, and cool it quickly on ice or in a refrigerator.
- Cook thoroughly, as soon as possible.

✦ Store fresh shellfish in an open container and under a damp towel to maintain humidity; keep in the refrigerator. Never store cockles, large butter, or horse clams in water for more than two hours because they'll die and spoil. However, Native littlenecks and Manila clams should be purged in cold seawater for at least 4 hours. Maximum storage times vary, so consult the health department websites.

**8. Know how to cook your shellfish.** Consult the state health department website for current advice on various ways to prepare shellfish (**doh.wa.gov**, search "shellfish cooking"). The Department of Health website also lists visual signs to let you know when your shellfish is thoroughly cooked.

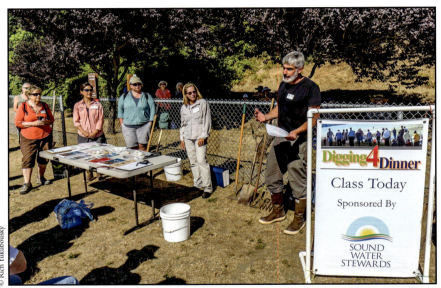

© Rich Yukubousky

*A Digging 4 Dinner class, given on Whidbey by Sound Water Stewards volunteers*

# If physical mobility is a challenge...

Don't let age, ability, or physical limitations prevent you from enjoying our beaches. Island County offers many beach opportunities whether you or a member of your party is in a wheelchair, pushing a stroller, using walking aids, or recovering from an injury. Here are some suggestions. For upland trail opportunities, see Barrier-free Trails, Chapter 6, pg. 169.

If you have difficulty getting down to the water's edge, the water's edge may come to you. This means knowing not only where but also when to go. Learn to read tide tables, and go to your destination when the tide is high; many beaches will be covered with water just feet from you, high and dry, sitting on a bench, watching from a patch of sand or grass, or standing in a parking lot.

A bonus in going out to high tides is that the best daytime high tides are in the winter, when you may be aching to get out of the house but not out into the cold. This is when those premier view parking spots are empty and available, and all you need to do to enjoy the smells and sounds of the sea is to open your window and take them in with your nose and ears.

## Parking spots, views, piers

The sites with premier parking views are listed in the Table of Shoreline Accesses (see pgs. 184–187) under Parking Vista. All parking spots in this category are open to anyone. Many disability parking spots have views too. Eligibility for disability parking is found at **dmv.org** under Qualifications for Disability License Plates and Placards.

And instead of getting near the water, why not get above it? Most piers, ramps, and docks are unstable and lack rails, but a few are sturdy and accessible all year long. Sturdy piers at both the Oak Harbor and Langley marinas lead to great viewing of boats and scenery. The Coupeville wharf offers exhibits on sea mammals and marine ecology, shops, restaurants, and frequent views of marine life in the waters below. The Clinton pier has great views, covered seating, and is easily reached through Clinton Beach Park. All of these have nearby restrooms with some degree of accessibility.

Remember that at floating docks, the steepness of the ramps to get to them is dependent on the height of the tide. High tide means a more level angle. Low tides may mean the ramps are far too steep to try, particularly with abrupt transitions onto the docks. Boat docks themselves do not have rails so having a companion along is advisable.

## Beaches with multiple accessible amenities

Some beaches have multiple accessible amenities close together, such as restrooms, picnic areas, good viewing of wildlife and scenery, and handicapped parking. These are some of the most accessible.

## Deception Pass State Park: West Beach (Site 1)

A meeting room, picnic table and grill, and a loop trail designed for accessibility are clustered in one area. Enter on the paved path to this area between the kiosks at the south end of the parking lot. The accessible-designated picnic table and grill sit on their own deck right against Cranberry Lake. Restrooms and easily-used picnic areas are nearby.

The Dunes Trail, a paved nature trail with interpretive signs, starts just beyond the meeting hall. Although intended for accessibility, tree roots have pushed up parts of the trail, so persons with assistive devices may not be able to travel the whole loop. Detours have been created on the level firm ground beside some of these obstacles but not all. However, the most spectacular part of this trail, reached by taking the right fork, is easily accessible. There is boardwalk through grass-covered dunes and a view of a remarkable Douglas fir more than 800 years old, astonishingly and curvaceously shaped by the elements (see photo pg. 22).

Off the north end of the West Beach parking lot are picnic tables and grassy, level viewing areas that look north across the waters as they flow to and from the Deception Pass Bridge. Designated parking spots offer views and parking for ADA compliant restrooms. The restrooms are a bit of an uphill climb from the parking, so wheelchair users may need some help to reach them.

Numerous picnic areas with tables, and some with grills, are scattered along the entire west end of the large parking lot. These are near the beach, close to parking, and reasonably near ADA retrofitted restrooms.

## Cornet Bay and Hoypus Point (Sites 2-4)

Cornet Bay has a mix of private and public facilities. Encountered first on the left is a public county dock, then a privately owned store and marina, and lastly the state park lands with a public boat launch and recreation area, which are part of Deception Pass State Park. The large, clean, ADA compliant restrooms near the boat launch serve the entire area and also offer an ADA friend-ly shower and ADA parking. Accessible picnic areas with grills are scattered nearby and at the marina store. A shelter with two tables near the ADA parking and restrooms offers overhead cover and can be reserved for group events. The nearby boat launch offers a viewing bench and interpretive signs.

The nearby mile-long Hoypus Point trail is paved, wide, and flat and is accessible to most persons with disabilities. At the trail entrance is a locked gate with a paved, 36-inch wide bypass that makes a tight curve around the far left post and also drops off sharply at its edge. Persons in hand-powered wheelchairs are advised that it can be negotiated but should be done so only with an assistant. Longer-length motorized chairs will be unable to make this turn. More information on this trail is on pg. 174.

## Oak Harbor Town Beaches and Marina (Sites 11-14)

The entire Oak Harbor waterfront is fully accessible, including several ADA compliant restrooms, paths, kitchen shelters, picnic areas, playground, and other amenities. One can negotiate from one end to the other on the wide and level paths, some with foot-level lighting.

However, it's a long walk or wheel from Flintstone Park to the fascinating Oak Harbor Marina, so it may be easier to drive to the marina, just below Skagit Valley College, and park in the marina's large lot. The marina docks are sturdy concrete and fully accessible via a solid pier and ramp with railings. The connector plate between the ramp and concrete dock is less abrupt than those at most other docks. Platforms set out over the water at the end offer your own picnic table with wide views of water and sky past the boats. For those who love boats, there are hours of fun and exploration to be had.

## Fort Casey State Park and Keystone Jetty (Sites 29 and 30)

Near the fort, there is no parking close to the water, but the panoramic views are spectacular. The most striking views are from the lighthouse area, especially from parking spots along the road. Persons who are relatively mobile can negotiate the hard-packed and level grass, which leads from the turning circle below the lighthouse to views above the beach. There is no parking on the loop, so a driver would drop off passengers and park nearby. ADA compliant restrooms and parking are down at the fort parking lot where an ADA trail leads to the fort. (See pg. 177.)

At the Keystone Jetty state parking lot next to the Coupeville-Port Townsend ferry, parking spots above the beach have panoramic views facing Admiralty Inlet. This is a great place to watch winter storms, sea birds, and the comings and goings of the ferry, and there are ADA accessible restrooms.

## South Whidbey Harbor at Langley (Site 50)

The small park here offers picnic tables, including one with room for a wheelchair, ADA accessible restrooms, easily negotiated paved surfaces, and views across the marina to Camano Island and the Cascade mountains. The top level of the marina pier is also wheelchair accessible and offers panoramic views. The view from the upper pier down onto the visiting sailboats is delightful. However, the ramps down to the boat docks are steep with abrupt transition plates onto the docks and they lack full safety railings, so they should probably be avoided.

## Clinton Beach Park (Site 54)

Clinton Beach Park is the first universal access beach in Washington state, meaning it exceeds ADA guidelines to be more accessible to persons for whom ADA standards are not enough. Visitors at Clinton Beach Park can now walk or wheel to, or very near to, the summer high tide mark. Standard wheelchairs, walkers, canes, crutches, wagons, strollers, and other assistive devices can easily navigate the bright blue mats to get as close as possible to the water's edge (see photos pgs. 98 and 182). These mats have a darker edge to be more visible to persons with visual impairment. Note that because of high beach erosion by winter storms, these mats are removed and stored from mid-October to mid-May of the following year.

Other improvements to accessibility have been made through joint efforts of the South Whidbey Port District and Island Beach Access, which wants to do similar projects on other island beaches. Two extra-wide, ecologically friendly handicapped parking spaces make it easier to get in and out of vehicles. Paved accesses serve two separate picnic areas, one covered by a living roof (green roof), and the other with interpretive signs overlooking the beach and pier. Each has a table with wheelchair space. The restrooms are ADA compliant. A children's play area can be reached easily over a hard-packed surface.

A gentle ramp leads from the park's open picnic area to the sturdy and fully accessible Clinton pier, which offers covered shelter from which you can enjoy views of water, wildlife, and and the comings and goings of the Clinton-Mukilteo ferry.

### English Boom Historical Preserve (Site 58)

With panoramic views to Mount Baker and the Cascades, this site has designated disability parking that gives easy wheelchair access up to a short walkway and viewing platform. A ramp leads up to an open-sided shelter with a picnic table. The preserve has a salt marsh, mud flats, beach berm, a nearby heron rookery providing habitat for multiple bird species and occasional seals on the beach. There is no restroom. (See pg. 171.)

### Camano Island and Cama Beach State Park (Sites 66 and 65)

Camano Island State Park has an accessible enclosed kitchen shelter next to the beach, as well as accessible campsites and tourist cabin in the campground. There are six accessible restrooms, including two at the boat launch. To reserve campsites, the cabin, or the kitchen shelter call 360-387-3031 or go to the Washington State Parks website, **parks.wa.gov**.

At nearby Cama Beach Historic State Park, visitors who can document their handicapped status can rent their choice of two historic fishing cabins, both retrofitted with accessible bathrooms. Also accessible are historic buildings that house a camp store, a wooden boat center, and up the hill, the Cama Center, including a cafe, meeting rooms, and bathrooms, all fully accessible. Another ADA restroom is at the drop-off shelter where people wait for a shuttle bus to take them to the cabins at the beach level or to the Cama Center. Persons renting accessible cabins should contact the Park Office at 360-387-1550 to arrange ahead for an escort to the parking spot adjacent to each cabin.

These are the only private cars allowed to drive or park in the cabin area. For online information and reservations, go the Washington State Parks website.

### Other accessible beach experiences: Explore for your favorites

*Many other Island County beaches offer some degree of accessibility. Taking time to explore beaches may reveal those with special delights for you.*

### Sounds and smells

**Hastie Lake Boat Launch (Site 18)**

On stormy high tide days, lofty waves break on the rock wall with the white spray and noise we expect only on the outer coast.

**Libbey Beach Park (Site 20)**

The receding tide makes music in the stones of the pebble beach below. Offshore here is the largest kelp forest in all of Washington State. It is part of the Smith and Minor Islands Aquatic Reserve, and you'll find interpretive signs in two languages.

### Dramatic views

**Ebey's Landing (Site 28)**

Enjoy the near-infinite view through the Strait with no land between you and Asia.

**Double Bluff Beach (Site 44)**

Water hits the wall at high tides, and the view of waves crossing Useless Bay is awe-inspiring. At low tides the sheer expanse of sand is impressive, and the power of water and wind are evident in the magnificent bluffs nearby.

**English Boom Preserve (Site 58)**

Across and beyond Skagit Bay, the Cascade mountain range and Mount Baker appear very close on clear days.

**Livingston Bay (Site 62)**

Directly south, Mount Rainier is framed by Kayak Point on the mainland and the south end of Camano Island. To the east is a view of the Stillaguamish River.

**Camano Island State Park (Site 66)**

Sited directly across from Holmes Harbor are views of Whidbey Island, Baby Island, and the Olympic mountains.

### Privacy and quiet

**Dugualla Bay Preserve (Site 7)**

Park on the shoulder here and take in the rich and varied habitats with wetlands, a grassy dike, and mudflats.

### Glendale Beach (Site 55)

Enjoy the views here across Saratoga Passage, including trains, ferries, and sometimes whales.

### English Boom Preserve (Site 58)

Share the quiet open spaces here with eagles, herons, and sometimes at low tides, seals resting on the beach.

### Livingston Bay (Site 62)

The beauty here is the empty, spacious, infinite view to the south, on some days flooded with light.

*Space for family and friends*

Especially beloved for large gatherings are **West Beach** at Deception Pass State Park, **Windjammer Park** at the Oak Harbor Waterfront, **Fort Casey State Park, Double Bluff Beach, Dave Mackie Park** at Maxwelton Beach, and **Camano Island State Park**. For these and more, look at the Table of Shoreline Accesses (see pgs. 184-187) for areas with accessible restrooms as well as picnic tables, grills, playgrounds, and even swimming.

*Did you find...*
1. *Stairs*
2. *Rocks*
3. *Pebbles*
4. *Log*
5. *Loose sand*
6. *Steep access*

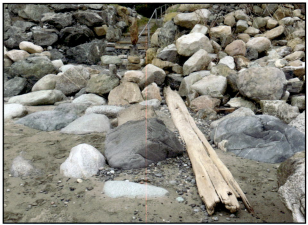

© Jeanie McElwain

*How many barriers to accessibility can you find?*

*Share and increase accessibility*

Follow the work of Sound Water Stewards and other organizations, such as Island Beach Access and Friends of Camano Island Parks, and your local port and park districts. Join in their efforts to increase accessibility on our beaches and trails up to or beyond the ADA-recommended guidelines. See Chapter 6 on Trails for other organizations that would appreciate your help in making the beautiful public lands and beaches of Whidbey and Camano Islands available to all of us, whatever our ability levels.

# SWS Coordinators' favorite beaches for children

## CAMANO ISLAND

**Iverson Spit Preserve (Site 63)**

Children and adults enjoy climbing on driftwood and piling it up into shelters. Bury your feet or body in sand on the long beach. Wade or swim in the shallow warm water. Don't miss the short walk across a field to the very special Hobbit Trail. No drinking water is available, but there is a portable toilet.

**Camano Island State Park (Site 66)**

Enjoy miles of shoreline, driftwood to play on, and picnic tables right on the beach. By the upper parking lot is an excellent interpretive trail: a half mile loop with over a dozen look-and-learn stations identifying trees, plants, and habitat.

## WHIDBEY ISLAND

**Dave Mackie Park (Site 52)**

Enjoy a nice sandy beach, lots of driftwood, a playground, and restrooms.

**Freeland Park (Site 41)**

This wonderful beach offers a covered picnic area, playground, and restrooms. Look for signage before entering the water; there have been some issues with contamination. Noctiluca (sea sparkle) blooms at the end of the summer, so bring a stick to the dock after dark and stir the water to watch it bioluminesce.

**Double Bluff Beach (Site 44)**

Here there is warm shallow water for swimming, skim boarding, and paddle boarding, or spend the day playing in the sand. This beach is also an off-leash dog park, with a foot rinse station and restrooms.

**Langley Seawall Park (Site 49)**

In spring, see gray whales in Saratoga Passage; also visit the Langley Whale Center at 117 Anthes Ave. Explore the waterfront's intertidal area for marine life, but be careful on the mud flats; kids can sink and lose their boots in the mud. Public restrooms are a short walk away.

**Ebey's Landing (Site 28)**

Great hiking and beach walking, but bring coats to fight the cold wind. The Jacob Ebey House is always a hit. There is a vault toilet, but no water.

**Fort Casey State Park (Site 29)**

Explore the old fort (ideally with a flashlight) and the lighthouse, take beach hikes, and fly kites on the huge lawn. There are picnic tables and full facilities.

**Joseph Whidbey State Park (Site 16)**

This popular park includes accessible parking; playfield; easy two-mile loop hike through forest; wetland and grassland habitats; and a long pebbly beach for exploring marine life. Bring jackets for the cold wind. At times, Navy jets soaring overhead can be entertaining and noisy.

# Make your dog dance for joy

Dogs are a big part of the island lifestyle. They welcome visitors to shops, fetch sticks at the beach, keep a watchful eye on the farm, and panhandle treats at the drive-up. They love a good time and give joy generously. Many an islander owes the better part of a daily fitness program to canine best friends who make exercise fun. So take your dog with you. Always clean up after your pet no matter where they happen to poop (see pg. 118).

## OFF-LEASH DOG PARKS

One way to enjoy a day in Island County is to take your best friend to one of the off-leash parks. FETCH! (Free Exercise Time for Canines and their Humans) works with the county parks department to promote and maintain some of the parks listed below.

**Technical Drive Off-leash Dog Park,** 501 Technical Dr, Oak Harbor.

From Hwy 20 turn N on Goldie Rd for 1 mile, then E on Technical Dr. The fenced park, just over an acre in size, is on R at the street's end.

**Clover Valley Off-leash Area,** 799 Ault Field Rd, Oak Harbor.

From Hwy 20 go W on Ault Field Rd approximately 1 mile. The entrance to this 3-acre, fully fenced dog park is on R, just past the intersection with Oak Harbor Rd, W of the Clover Park ball fields. This park is maintained by the residents using it, so pack out everything you bring. If you use this site, consider joining the monthly cleaning meeting to keep the park in good shape.

**Patmore Pit,** 530 Patmore Rd, Coupeville.

Patmore Pit is S of Coupeville, W of the Naval Air Station Outlying Field. From Hwy 20, turn onto Patmore Rd. Take second road on L, a short lane with dog park entrance gate at the end. Site includes 15 fully-fenced acres of open space and woods. Find a separate fenced agility area by following a path straight back from parking area.

**Greenbank Farm,** 765 Wonn Rd, Greenbank.

This park, one of the largest off-leash parks on Whidbey Island, is just N of Greenbank. Although open to the public, this site is also a working farm, so you must have good control of your dog to prevent interaction with waterfowl and livestock. One entrance is at the retail area of Greenbank Farm; another is farther N at the parking area just off Hwy 525. Be sure to obey the signs that designate where the off-leash begins and where you must leash up again.

**Double Bluff Beach Access,** south end of Double Bluff Rd (Site 44).

This site offers great beach walking. The off-leash area starts at the windsock, about 500 feet from the parking lot. *Note: Owners allowing their dogs to run off-leash before this point are subject to a $500 fine for violating the county leash law.*

A dog-height drinking fountain and dog rinse station are provided next to the parking lot. Parking can be tight, especially on summer weekends. Don't park illegally; you risk being towed. In this multi-use area, respect the off-leash boundaries, and pick up after your dogs! Your dog can explore large pieces of driftwood, sand dunes, and water access. Keep dogs safe and off the bluff.

**Marguerite Brons Memorial Park,** 2837 Becker Rd, Clinton.

From Hwy 525, turn S on Bayview Rd. The park entrance is about 0.5 mile on your L, a short distance past the cemetery. Follow gravel road to parking area. This 13-acre park is completely fenced with three zones: a two-acre open meadow play area with a covered picnic shelter and water station; a small-dog area; and two gates leading to a wooded area with trails to explore.

**Henry Hollow Dog Park,** 876 West Camano Dr, Camano Island.

From Terry's Corner go S on East Camano Dr. In 2.5 miles turn R onto North Camano Hill Rd. In 3.3 miles turn L onto West Camano Dr; the park is on R. This 7-acre dog park is the only designated off-leash area for dogs on Camano Island. Two fenced areas are available, one for larger dogs and one for smaller. Parking is limited. Dogs must be on leash until you're within the fenced-in areas.

**Heritage Park,** 9800 276th St NW, Stanwood.

From Hwy 532 turn N onto 102nd Ave NW, travel 0.4 mile, turn E on 276th St NW/Lovers Rd, and in 0.4 mile Heritage Park is on the R. Stanwood's off-leash dog park is part of the larger Heritage Park.

### *Good citizenship will keep opportunities open*

As the islands grow more crowded, dog owners' courtesy and good citizenship grow more important in keeping opportunities open to pets and owners, including dog parks. FETCH! asks owners to diligently observe these practices:

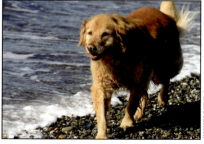

© Dan Pederson

- ✦ Use plastic bags to clean up after your dog anywhere they poop.
- ✦ Keep your dog from digging holes.
- ✦ Stop bothersome behavior immediately.
- ✦ Keep your dog on leash until in the designated area.
- ✦ Be respectful of all users of the park.
- ✦ Never allow dogs to interact with or harass wildlife.
- ✦ Spay or neuter your dog.
- ✦ Learn and follow dog licensing laws: see islandcountywa.gov

Contact FETCH! at fetchparks.org for more information about dog parks.

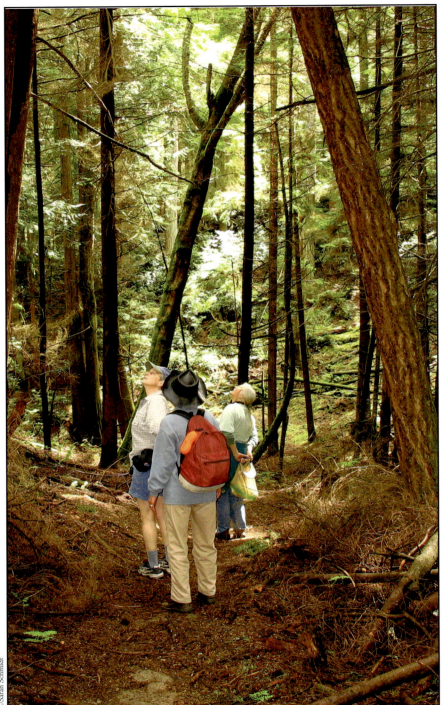

©Sarah Schmidt

# CHAPTER SIX

## Guide to Trails

Whidbey and Camano Islands offer miles of public use trails on shoreline, prairie, and forest lands. They're maintained by either state, national, or county park systems; school districts and municipalities; or private non-profit organizations. Please treat these trails with respect: observe any rules, clean up after your pets, and pick up litter. As of 2020, dogs on leash are allowed unless otherwise noted.

The following descriptions provide general information about locations offering upland walking trails. Trail maps aren't included because trails change often. Research a site before you go. Apps and websites offer crowd-sourced maps, but cell phones may not receive signals at all locations. When maps are posted at the trailhead, take a photograph for reference during your hike.

### Barrier-free Trails

Few Island County trails are completely barrier free, but some come close. References marked with the International Access Symbol describe popular upland trails considered accessible for most mobility-challenged persons. Details about accessible beaches are in Chapter 5, pages 159-164.

### Some resources on Island County trails

**Crandell, Maribeth with Hartt, Jack.** *Hiking Close to Home: Whidbey, Fidalgo, and Guemes Islands.* 2019. Trail descriptions with maps and information about public transit access. At local bookstores and **hikingclosetohome.weebly.com**.

**Friends of Camano Island Parks (FOCIP).** *Walking the Camano Island Trails.* Maps, directions, elevations, history and more about Camano Island trails. Revised regularly and sold locally. FOCIP is an all-volunteer, nonprofit organization that stewards the state and county parks on Camano Island. Their guided walks schedule is at **friendsofcamanostateparks.org**.

**Hartt, Jack.** *Exploring Deception Pass: An Insider's Guide to Washington's Favorite State Park.* 2016. Descriptions of major trails, photos, natural history, and accessibility levels at major facilities and some trails. See **deceptionpass-foundation.org**.

Websites don't always provide comprehensive trail maps, and the capacity to print maps off the sites varies. You may want to explore multiple online sources to find the information that suits you best.

- **All Trails**, alltrails.com. Good online maps for most trails in Island County. Directions, trail length, elevation variations, and amenities. Enlarge elevation maps to see exact trail names and lengths; reduce to get better views of geography and roadways. Users must create an account and pay a fee to print maps. An app is also available.
- **Washington Trails Association**, wta.org. The nation's largest statewide trails association, dedicated to protecting Washington's trails. Includes excellent trail maps.
- **Whidbey Island Trails**, whidbeyislandtrails.org. A collaborative site built by users and specializing in mapping connections between separate trail systems.

## The trails

Trail locations are shown by their letter designation on the Site Map, pages 188-189. These trails are owned and managed by the organizations listed below, identified at the end of each trail description.

- Camano Senior Services Association–**camanocenter.org**
- City of Oak Harbor–**oakharborwa.org**
- Coupeville Port District–**portoc.org**
- Earth Sanctuary–**earthsanctuary.org**
- Friends of Camano Island Parks–**friendsofcamanoislandparks.org**
- Island County Parks & Trails–**islandcounty.gov/PublicWorks/Parks**
- Meerkerk Rhododendron Gardens–**meerkerkgardens.org**
- National Park System (Ebey's Landing National Historical Reserve)–**nps.gov,** maps at **wta.org**
- Oak Harbor Garry Oak Society–**ohgarryoaksociety.org**
- Pacific Rim Institute for Environmental Studies (PRI)–**pacificriminstitute.org**
- South Whidbey Parks & Recreation District–**swparks.org**
- South Whidbey Port District–**portofsouthwhidbey.com**
- South Whidbey School District–**sw.wednet.edu**
- The Whidbey Institute–**whidbeyinstitute.org**
- Washington State Parks–**parks.wa.gov**
- Whidbey Camano Land Trust–**wclt.org**. (Check website for updates about new preserves)
- Whidbey Watershed Stewards–**whidbeywatersheds.org**

# Camano Island Trails

## ♿ A. English Boom Preserve (Site 58)

The accessible trail boardwalk, destroyed in a storm, wasn't fully replaced. It's now a wheelchair-accessible viewing platform with views of Mount Baker and Skagit Bay. ADA designated parking is near the ramps to the accessible viewing platform and covered picnic shelter. The foot trail behind the shoreline, closed in winter, isn't ADA compliant, but some people using canes are able to use the trail in dry weather. (Island County Parks)

*Follow directions to Site 58, pg. 103.*

## ♿ B. Camano Center

This ¼-mile trail, gravel in some parts and bark in others, leads through meadow, forest, and a legacy garden. Officially ADA compliant, but soft bark and size of loose gravel make it difficult for some persons pushing wheelchairs. (Camano Senior Services Association)

*From Terry's corner, follow East Camano Drive for 1 mile, then turn R onto Cross Island Rd and immediately get into the righthand lane. Turn R on Arrowhead Rd, and R on the driveway toward the school, then L into the parking lot for the Camano Center.*

## C. Kristoferson Creek

Visit Camano Island's largest salmon-bearing stream, with three kinds of salmon documented (see box pgs. 112-113). A short trail includes a spot to view wildlife within the 10 acres of protected riparian and wetland habitat. (Whidbey Camano Land Trust)

*From Terry's Corner, go S on East Camano Dr for 2 miles. Turn L onto Russell Rd and after a long block, turn L on Sapphire Dr. The first cross street is David St; just before you reach it, on L you'll see a field with a small sign. Park on the road shoulder. A short trail leads to an information kiosk, a bridge, and a viewing platform. From the kiosk, there is also a short trail, under ½ mile, to Cedar Grove.*

## D. Camano Ridge Forest Preserve

Near the highest point of Camano Island, multiple trails wind through 400 acres of forested uplands. As one of the largest continuous properties on Camano Island, the preserve provides critical wildlife habitat. Many trails include short, steep climbs, but Road Trail, an old logging road, has a fairly even surface and gradual hills. Hike, mountain bike, or ride a horse. Hunting is allowed in the preserve in season. (Island County Parks)

*For Can Ku entrance: From Terry's Corner follow East Camano Dr to Can Ku Rd. Follow Can Ku Rd up the hill to a small entrance on R. For Camano Ridge entrance: From Terry's Corner follow East Camano Dr and turn R onto Cross Island Rd (traffic light). After about 2 miles, turn L on North Camano Ridge Rd and in 0.9 mile a large parking lot and the trailhead will be on your L, just before Carp Lake.*

## E. Iverson Spit Preserve (Site 63)

Enjoy flat trails through 120 acres of fields and beach grasses with views of Mount Baker and the Cascades. Beach and viewing platform are nearby. (Island County Parks)

*Follow directions to Site 63, pg. 111.*

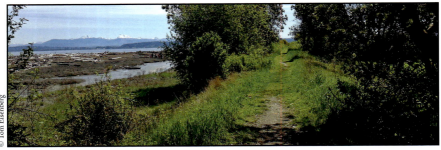

*Iverson Spit Trail*

### F. Barnum Point County Park (Site 68)

Walk over 2½ miles of trails through mature forest, open meadows, and marsh. A viewing platform, midpoint on the Bluff Trail, provides two benches with sweeping views of the Cascade mountains, Port Susan, Puget Sound, Camano Island south to Camano Head, and Mount Rainier. Two beach accesses lead to a mile of beach, primarily below high bluffs on Port Susan Bay. (Island County Parks)

*Follow directions to Site 68, pg. 121.*

### G. Four Springs Lake Preserve

This venue for weddings, meetings, conferences, and shows includes picnic facilities, restrooms, and trails through 50 acres of woodlands and meadow. (Island County Parks)

*585 Lewis Lane. From Hwy 532 drive S on East Camano Drive. Turn R on Camano Hill Rd, and in 1 mile turn R onto Lewis Lane.*

### H. Elger Bay Preserve and Nature Trail

This park, next to Elger Bay Elementary School, supports students and has a Community Wildlife Habitat demonstration garden. Enjoy 170 acres of riparian and scrub habitats with trails, an informational kiosk, a 1-mile nature trail loop with signage, and a beaver marsh with viewing platform and benches. The trails are generally easy to walk. (Island County Parks)

*From Hwy 532 drive S on East Camano Dr for 5.8 miles. At intersection with Monticello, continue straight 1.2 miles on Elger Bay Rd, turn R onto Dry Lake Rd and park on the shoulder on either side of road.*

### I. Cama Beach Historical State Park (Site 65)

These 486 acres offer multiple trails, including loop trails with viewing platforms, views from the bluff, paths along waterfront and through forest, and Cranberry Lake Trail, a 2-mile round trip through forest to a beaver lake. The Cross Island Trail to Camano Island State Park provides another 2 miles of round trip hiking. (WA State Parks)

*Follow directions to Site 65, pg. 114.*

### J. Camano Island State Park (Site 66)

This camping park offers 6,700 feet of rocky shoreline and beach with views of Saratoga Passage, the Olympic Mountains, and Mount Rainier. Find multiple trails within the 244 acres to explore the beach, marsh, forest, and bluff rim. The Al Emerson Nature trail is family-friendly; use the brochure identifying trees and other plants. (WA State Parks)

*Follow directions to Site 66, pg. 116.*

## Whidbey Island Trails

### North Whidbey

### K. Goose Rock / Deception Pass State Park (Site 1)

The park includes 40 miles of trails on both Whidbey and Fidalgo Islands. Reach Goose Rock by crossing under Deception Pass bridge, either from the parking lot at the bridge's southern end or from North Beach. Multiple trails

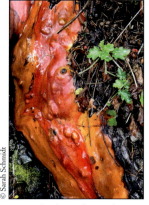

provide more than 2 miles of hiking. The Perimeter Trail circles Goose Rock and provides views of Deception Pass, Ben Ure Island, and Cornet Bay. The Goose Rock Summit trail ends at 484 ft elevation. Near the summit is the area called "the Balds," an environmentally sensitive site scraped to bedrock by receding glaciers 11,000 years ago. The site now features thin layers of soil and unique native plants. Avoid walking on the fragile meadows. Visit the west summit for views of the Strait of Juan de Fuca, the San Juan Islands, and Naval Air Station Whidbey Island. Training flights for Navy jets are sometimes loud. (WA State Parks)

*Bark of Pacific madrone tree on Goose Rock Perimeter Trail*

*Follow directions to Site 1, pg. 21. From entry kiosk follow signs to North Beach.*

### K2. Sand Dunes Interpretive Trail, Deception Pass State Park

Reached from the south end of the West Beach parking lot, this paved, ¾-mile loop nature trail is buckled by tree roots in some places; this may prevent some people with assistive devices from completeing the whole loop. The right fork offers a smooth path to a spectacular Douglas fir twisted with age and time (see photo pg. 22). More information on this trail is on pg. 160.

*Follow directions to Site 1, pg. 21. From entry kiosk follow signs to West Beach/Cranberry Lake.*

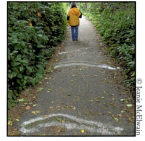

*Tree roots blocking Sand Dunes trail*

**L. Hoypus Point, Deception Pass State Park (Site 4)**

Miles of upland trails lead through the best area on north Whidbey for huge old growth Douglas fir, western red cedar, and big leaf maple. Formerly logged areas are re-growing a young forest. (WA State Parks)

*Follow directions to Site 4, pg. 26. Foot traffic only at Cornet Bay Rd trailhead for Hoypus Point Natural Forest Area; take Ducken Rd to Hoypus Hill trailhead for walkers, mountain bikers, and equestrians.*

**L2. Hoypus Point Accessible Trail**

The marked start of this 1-mile trail, at the northeast end of the Cornet Bay parking lot, has accessible features including handicapped parking and an ADA bathroom. The trail from the parking lot was a road leading to the old ferry landing that serviced the area before the bridge was built. Erosion forced closure to vehicles, leaving a flat, paved trail easy to walk through magnificent stands of trees. Accessible benches provide scenic views of the Deception Pass Bridge. The trail ends with views of Fidalgo, Hope, Skagit, and Kiket Islands. More information for wheelchair users is on pg. 160.

**M. Dugualla State Park (Site 8)**

To prevent logging, state parks acquired this area in 1992. Several miles of trails wind through deeply shaded, conifer forest and open alder groves. A steep trail with switchbacks through moss-covered big-leaf maples leads to the beach. Note the location of the well-hidden trail entrance and then enjoy a mile of beach walking. Enjoy over 4 miles of walking and about 600 feet elevation gain on a loop of the outer trails. (WA State Parks, managed as a satellite of Deception Pass State Park in collaboration with Island County)

*Follow directions to Site 8, pg. 31.*

**N. Oak Harbor Waterfront Trail (Sites 11-14)**

Three miles of paved trail parallels the waterfront from the city marina, through Windjammer Park (with multiple amenities for families and children), and west to upper beach grass habitat, much by way of a boardwalk with night lighting. All facilities are accessible. More trail information is on pg. 161. (City of Oak Harbor)

*Follow directions to Sites 11-14, pgs. 37-42.*

**O. Garry Oak Tree Tour, Oak Harbor**

This 3-mile, self-guided walking tour highlights the Garry oak, *Quercus garryana*, Oak Harbor's namesake tree and the only native oak in Washington State. Many heritage oaks are estimated at 150 to 300 years old. The tour celebrates oak trees on public and private property; respect private property and don't trespass. The Garry oak, once common on dry, open sites from British Columbia to California, forms a distinct meadow ecosystem with camas, shooting star, and other native plants and grasses. The ecosystem is critically imperiled; some areas of the Northwest have lost up to 99% of Garry oak habitat.

The tour winds through old town Oak Harbor, including Smith Park, the only park in the state composed completely of Garry oak trees. A Native Garden pocket park with interpretive signage is at the Oak Harbor Post Office where a 330-year-old oak was lost in 2014. (Oak Harbor Garry Oak Society)

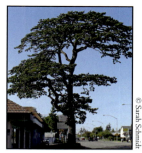

*Garry oak*

*Find the tour map available online as a PDF and as a brochure, published by the Oak Harbor Chamber of Commerce. Park at Sites 12-14 (pgs. 38-42) or somewhere in the tour area.*

### P. Beach View Farm Trail, Oak Harbor

Enjoy 1½ miles of trail connecting forest and farm to the beach. A Whidbey Camano Land Trust easement in 2016 protected the 315-acre Beach View Farm. With open fields and forest in the background, you can enjoy a foreground view of Swan Lake and the Strait of Juan de Fuca. The trail skirts a working farm—no dogs allowed. (Whidbey Camano Land Trust)

*The trail can be accessed at one end from West Beach Vista (Site 17) off West Beach Rd in Oak Harbor and at the other end at the parking lot of the Christian Reformed Church, 1411 Wieldraayer Rd, off of Swantown Rd. A map is on the WCLT website.*

### Q. Joseph Whidbey State Park (Site 16)

Several miles of trails wend along the beach and past a cattail marsh, with a 1-mile loop through forest and field. (WA State Parks)

*Follow directions to Site 16, pg. 43.*

### R. Del Fairfax Preserve, Oak Harbor

Dr. George Fairfax donated this 50-acre property to honor the memory of his wife, Del. It's maintained as wildlife habitat. A 1¼-mile trail includes a forest section and meadow loop with a bench. (Whidbey Camano Land Trust)

*1817 Zylstra Rd. From Highway 20 turn N onto Zylstra Rd. Continue for about 3 miles until the Zylstra Road Fire Station is on your L. Turn L onto a wide gravel road in front of the fire station. Park on the R next to the fence. Don't block the gravel road or the Fire Station bay doors.*

## CENTRAL WHIDBEY

### S. Fort Ebey State Park (Site 21)

Enjoy 25 miles of mixed-use walking and mountain biking trails in forest and on the bluff with peek-a-boo views of Admiralty Inlet and Olympic Mountains. Explore historic gun emplacements and underground rooms, open fields, and beach walking. Site is linked to the Kettles Trail System. (WA State Parks)

*Follow directions to Site 21, pg. 50.*

### T. Kettles Trail System, Coupeville

Kettles are depressions left from the receding glacier and are readily visible on the LIDAR map (see pg. 134). An up-to-date map is recommended to navigate the more than 35 miles of tangled trails. Find maps via the app Avenza pdf Maps, from Island County Parks, and a printed or online Trails Map from Ebey's Landing National Historical Reserve. You can also photograph the maps at trailhead kiosks. (Island County Parks)

*Begin at Fort Ebey State Park (Site 21, pg. 50) or park at one of the pullouts off Hwy 20 south of Libbey Rd.*

## U. Ebey's Bluff, Pratt Loop, Coupeville

The Pratt Loop trail skirts agricultural fields and enters the forest by the old Pratt sheep barn. Enjoy the forest and the understory of ocean spray (*Holodiscus discolor*). Emerge to views of Mount Baker, Mount Rainier, and across Ebey's Prairie to Admiralty Inlet. Return to the parking area or follow Ebey's Prairie Ridge Trail to reach Ebey's Bluff loop trail (see Site 28, pg. 61).

From here you can also walk a short distance to the historic Jacob and Sarah Ebey House and the Ebey Blockhouse, open to the public during the summer months; check with Ebey's Landing National Historical Reserve for details. A vault toilet is next to the parking area. The historic Sunnyside Cemetery is also interesting. (Partnership of the National Park Service, WA State Parks, Island County, and Town of Coupeville)

*Turn W off Hwy 20 onto Sherman Rd and continue straight on Cemetery Rd to the end. Park on the L at the Prairie Overlook opposite the far end of the cemetery, or continue between hedges to additional parking and Ebey's Reserve Trail Portal kiosk. The Pratt Loop Trail and Ebey's Prairie Ridge Trail start here.*

## V. Admiralty Inlet Natural Area Preserve, Coupeville

The Preserve includes 86 acres of old growth forest, rare prairie remnant, and bluff-top views. In May, the endangered prairie plant golden paintbrush (*Castilleja levisecta*), blooms. Douglas fir, grand fir, western hemlock, Pacific yew, Sitka spruce, and red alder trees stand along the 2½ mile loop trail. Many trees are more than 145 years old. (Whidbey Camano Land Trust)

*From Hwy 20, turn S at Coupeville traffic light onto S Main St, which beyond Terry Rd becomes S Engle Rd. Past Hill Rd, just after Engle Rd bends to the L, is a small gravel parking area on the L, before the houses. Park here and cross the road to the Preserve entrance.*

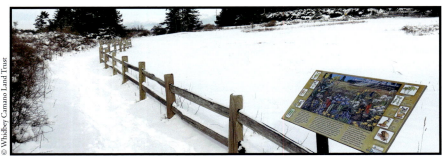

*Admiralty Preserve*

## W. Fort Casey Historical State Park (Sites 29-31)

This 999-acre park has 2 miles of beach on Admiralty Inlet, including Keystone Spit and nearly 2 miles of hiking trails. Also, explore the Admiralty Head Lighthouse and extensive historic fortifications. (WA State Parks)

*Follow directions to Sites 29-31, pgs. 63-66.*

### W2. Fort Casey ADA Loop

Follow directions to Site 29 and park near the ADA restroom in the main parking lot to access this ½-mile trail. A paved sidewalk leads to a packed gravel trail at the fort. Interpretive signs tell the fort's story, and a level, textured metal ramp leads to wide hallways and well-lit viewing rooms within the fort. The trail continues past bunkers, guns, and an ADA porta-potty, then climbs gently through forest on a hard-packed earth service road that ends at the park offices. Where the service road meets the paved park road, a steep incline and cement lip may hinder persons using wheelchairs or other devices; navigation may be easier at the exit south of the park building. Park offices are immediately to the left of the road into the Fort area, so accessibility can be checked out on the way into the Fort before deciding how much of the trail to attempt.

### X. Rhododendron/Kettles Trail, Coupeville

This 4-mile trail parallels Hwy 20. The Rhododendron section is from Rhododendron Park west to Main Street at the Coupeville traffic signal. The Kettles trail extends from Main St west to Winterhawk Lane where it joins the Kettles Trails complex. Completely paved and popular with all ages and abilities, the views are of prairie farmlands, mountains, and water. Most stanchion posts have been reset to make much of the trail accessible to wheelchairs. North of Broadway, the trail becomes hilly and could be a challenge for wheelchairs. (Island County Parks)

*Parking for either direction is available at the Coupeville Park and Ride at 201 S Main St. Parking is also available at Rhododendron Park.*

## Y. Rhododendron Park, Coupeville

Several trails loop through this heritage forest, recognized by the Washington Natural Heritage program as a rare remnant of a "...Douglas fir/western hemlock/Pacific rhododendron/evergreen huckleberry forest association," a unique assemblage of plants and dependent species endemic to Puget Lowlands of Washington. This forest type has old-growth trees much smaller in diameter than typical old-growth because of the gravelly and excessively drained soils. The oldest

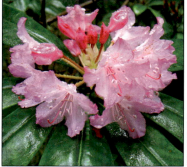

*Pacific rhododendron, the Washington state flower*

© Sarah Schmidt

Douglas firs here range from 270 to 350 years old. Many native rhododendrons in the understory are over 150 years old. Rhododendron Park is one of only five high-quality forest stands of this type left in the state.

Rhodie Road, running down the center for the length of the park, is now a paved trail closed to vehicles (see ADA trail below). (Island County Parks)

*North entrance: 20265 Hwy 20. Park entrance is about 1.5 miles from Patmore Rd going N, and 1.5 miles from Coupeville going S: Watch for the Park sign to Rhododendron Campground to find parking and access to the Rhododendron Park trail system. Campground is closed Nov-Apr but trails are open. South entrance: 502 W. Patmore Rd. From Hwy 20 turn W onto Patmore Rd; park entrance is about 0.5 mile on R. Here are athletic fields, full service restrooms, picnic area, picnic shelter, playground, and access to trail system. Vehicles may also park in pull-out 0.2 mile west of the main park entrance to access the bypass around the gate at the south end.*

### Y2. Rhododendron Park ADA Trail

An old chip-sealed road runs from the north parking lot off Hwy 20 and through this forested site to Patmore Rd on the south. Non-motorized travel only. Native rhododendrons flower May to June. The road is closed by gates from November to March; gate bypasses accommodate pedestrians and bicycles but are too narrow for some wheelchairs.

### Z. Pacific Rim Institute (Smith Prairie Reserve), Coupeville

The Prairie Reserve, on 175 acres, formerly was used as a state game farm. It includes a Douglas fir forest, remnant glacial outwash prairie, domestic fields converted to non-native grasses, and a homestead with several buildings. Efforts are focused on restoration of native prairie, Washington State's most rapidly disappearing and threatened ecosystem. In spring, the prairie blooms with endangered golden paintbrush, camas, chocolate lily, and others. The trail system is open for walking, pets on leash, and bicycles but no motorized vehicles. Prairie plants are rare and fragile; stay on the trails. (Pacific Rim Institute)

*180 Parker Rd. 3 miles S of Coupeville, exit Hwy 20 onto Morris Rd. Turn L almost immediately onto Parker Rd. Pacific Rim Institute (PRI) is 0.25 mile on R.*

## SOUTH WHIDBEY

### AA. Greenbank Farm, Greenbank

These 151 acres include 3 miles of trails, 12 acres of wetland, a bird watching platform, solar farm, Master Gardeners Demonstration Garden, playground, historic buildings, shops, art galleries, office space, and a large barn for community events. Enjoy views of the Cascades, Saratoga Passage, Admiralty Inlet, and Olympic Mountains. Trails meander through an open field, off-leash dog park and an on-leash forest loop. The forest area, county owned, allows for hunting in season. (Port of Coupeville)

*765 Wonn Rd. Turn off Hwy 525 onto Wonn Rd at the sign for Greenbank Farm, approximately 16 miles N of Clinton and 11 miles S of Coupeville. From Wonn Rd turn L* into Greenbank Farm parking lot. A secondary access point is a pullout about 0.5 mile N along Hwy 525 on E side of the road.

## BB. Meerkerk Rhododendron Gardens, Greenbank

This private, not-for-profit garden, open 9:00-4:00 daily except during high winds, has 10 acres of ornamental gardens and 43 acres of woodland with 4 miles of nature trails. Dogs must be leashed. Admission $5. (Meerkerk Gardens)

*3531 Meerkerk Ln. From Hwy 525, 2 miles S of Greenbank turn E onto Resort Rd. In 0.5 mile turn L onto Meerkerk Ln and follow signs to Visitor's Parking area.*

## CC. South Whidbey State Park, Freeland (Site 37)

Enjoy 3½ miles of trails through excellent stands of old-growth Douglas fir, Sitka spruce, western hemlock, and western red cedar, including one cedar over 500 years old. Some trails offer views of Admiralty Inlet and the Olympic Mountains. The beach access trail is closed indefinitely due to bluff erosion. (WA State Parks)

*Follow directions to Site 37, pg. 76.*

### ♿ CC2. South Whidbey State Park campground roads

The old campground is permanently closed to camping but open for daytime access. A paved road to the left of the restrooms slopes gently through former campgrounds to a small sedge-lined wetland. Here it meets a paved road, rich in varieties of forest and wetland plants, which leads left toward the Classic U old growth forest or right to return to the parking lot. This return, however, is blocked by a locked gate that chairs and scooters can't go around. Be cautioned also that the campground road can become slick from a build up of mud and dead leaves, so it may be best used in the dry season. The slope, though gentle, may be challenging to some persons using human-powered chairs.

## DD. Trillium Community Forest, Freeland

These 721 acres feature wildlife habitat, forested wetlands, and 7 miles of public trails (⅓ mile paved) to hike, bike, and horseback ride (where designated). The preserve is set up to protect and improve habitat; to that end, the trail system is designed to create large blocks of undisturbed forest for wildlife. For safety, there is no hiking, biking, or horseback riding during posted hunting seasons. (Whidbey Camano Land Trust)

*Hwy 525 Trailhead: Located just W of Hwy 525 off Pacific Dogwood Ln (0.9 miles N of Mutiny Bay Rd). Parking lot is for up to 12 passenger vehicles under 22'; trailer parking isn't allowed. Smugglers Cove Trailhead: One mile S of South Whidbey State Park, on the E side of Smugglers Cove Rd between Bald Eagle Way and Rhodie Ln. Parking lot accommodates horse trailers, buses, and RVs.*

### ♿ DD2. Trillium Community Forest ADA Loop

Accessible parking spots adjoin this ⅓-mile trail over hard-packed gravel and asphalt through mixed forest. Though titled "Level Loop," some slope may challenge those using human-powered wheelchairs. Total elevation change is 15 feet with a typical grade of 2%. The trail is closed to horses and bicycles.

*Bounty Loop Trailhead: Take Mutiny Bay Rd W from Hwy 525. Turn onto Bounty Loop Rd, L from the south and R from the north. Parking is at NW corner of Bounty Loop Rd. Parking lot holds 8 vehicles under 22 feet. Trailer parking not allowed.*

### EE. Freeland Wetland Preserve, Freeland

A ½-mile loop takes walkers by a wetland rich in plants and birds and through some upland forest. Interpretive signs explain how peat built up to create the wetland and how the waters move from this spot, through the ground, to Useless Bay. (Whidbey Watershed Stewards)

*From Hwy 525 turn toward Freeland on either Main or Scott. Where Main and Scott come together, turn NE on Newman Rd. Immediately past buildings on the R, turn R at Freeland Wetland Preserve sign.*

### FF. Earth Sanctuary, Langley

This privately-owned preserve offers 2 miles of trails through forested hills and past ponds and fens that display sculptures based on traditional labyrinths, standing stones, circles, and medicine wheels, plus a traditional Tibetan stupa. Open daily during daylight hours. Admission $7. No dogs. (Earth Sanctuary)

***Main entrance at 2059 Newman Rd, Langley:*** *From Hwy 525 turn N onto Double Bluff Rd (R from south, L from north). Turn R on Newman Rd to main entrance on L.* ***Second entrance to the arboretum and stupa*** *at 5536 Emil Rd, Langley. From Hwy 525, turn N onto Newman Rd (R from south, L from north). Turn R on Emil to entrance on L.*

### GG. Trustland Trails, Langley

These 200 acres of woodland, part of state trust lands since 1895, were transferred to South Whidbey Parks and Recreation in 2007 (through efforts by The Whidbey Camano Land Trust and others). A large, paved parking lot; picnic shelter; ½-mile ADA trail; and over 2 miles of multi-use loop trail are available. (South Whidbey Parks)

***From the south,*** *the Craw Rd entrance at Hwy 525 is somewhat blind, and is most safely reached by turning L off Hwy 525 at Maxwelton Rd, then R on Craw Rd to park entrance on L.* ***From the north,*** *if you miss the R onto Craw Rd, turn R onto Coles Rd and then R onto Craw.*

### GG2. Trustland Trails ADA Loop

This packed gravel, ½-mile loop is level, wide, and easy to navigate as it circles through primarily conifer forest. The large Trustland Trails parking area off Craw Rd is close to Hwy 525 and has handicapped spaces.

### HH. Saratoga Woods, Langley

Trails for hikers, mountain bikers, and equestrians abound in 120 wooded acres; included are a parking lot, picnic area, and portable toilet in season. Near the north end of the old airstrip, a trail to the west leads to Waterman Rock, a giant glacial erratic (a large boulder left by receding ice) that is 38 feet high and 60 feet long. (Island County Parks)

*4228 Saratoga Rd, Langley. From Hwy 525, turn N on Bayview Rd. Travel approximately 3 miles to DeBruyn Ave, turn L to stop sign and L on Saratoga Rd, continuing about 3 miles to park on L.*

## II. Putney Woods County Park, Langley

Enjoy 15 miles of trails in 600 acres of forest. Open for hikers, mountain bikers, and equestrians. This second-growth conifer forest has a native understory of salal, huckleberry, ferns, and mushrooms in season. The forest varies from relatively open to densely wooded, with mostly flat terrain and some steep-sided ravines. Three trail systems include Saratoga Woods Preserve, Putney Woods (formerly Goss Lake Woods), and Metcalf Trust. Carry a map or take a photo of the map at the trailhead kiosk. A portable toilet and parking for cars and trailers are available. (Island County Parks)

*From Hwy 525, go N on Bayview Rd 1.5 miles, L on Andreason Rd to stop sign, and R on Lone Lake Rd. Parking area is on R, 0.5 mile N of Keller Rd.*

## JJ. South Whidbey Elementary School Trails, Langley

This forested trail system, behind what is now the Elementary School, is open to the public on weekends and on weekdays when school is not in session. (South Whidbey School District)

*5380 Maxwelton Rd. From Hwy 525, go N on Maxwelton Rd 0.9 mile to sign on L for South Whidbey Elementary School. Park on N side of driveway next to kiosk or in school lots outside school hours. Trails start in the woods to the far right when facing the school.*

## KK. South Whidbey Community Park, Langley

Miles of groomed trails for hiking and biking, with multiple loop trails, offer easy to moderate walking. The park has a playground, skate park, picnic area, baseball and soccer fields, and restrooms. (South Whidbey Parks)

*5495 Maxwelton Rd entrance: From Hwy 525 turn N onto Maxwelton Rd, R from the south or L from the north. Entry road is just N of the high school, or R with well-marked sign. Trails can also be accessed from the Sports Complex entrance at 5598 Langley Rd.*

## KK2. South Whidbey Community Park accessible trails

Use the Maxwelton Road entrance to reach wide and mostly flat trails of packed gravel and hard earth. They wind through the forest and around the park facilities; pick whichever works best for you. The Waterman Loop brings you out downhill from the parking area, a long push uphill to the trailhead. Restrooms are accessible.

## LL. Maxwelton Nature Preserve, Clinton (Site 51)

This property, run by Whidbey Watershed Stewards and owned by a school district, is fully accessible. Packed earth trails and boardwalks lead ½-mile through the forest and past views of Maxwelton Creek. This is a classroom facility, so come when students aren't on site. (South Whidbey School District)

*Follow directions to Site 51, pg. 93.*

## MM. Waterman Shoreline Preserve, Langley

This paved walking and biking path through mature coastal forest was once a roadway connecting Bob Galbreath Rd and Wilkinson Rd. Except for this trail, the rest of the 59-acre preserve is closed, including 35 acres of protected tidelands extending 2,000 feet along Possession Sound. (Whidbey Camano Land Trust)

*Bob Galbreath Rd. From Hwy 525 just west of the Clinton ferry, turn N onto Bob Galbreath Rd. Waterman Preserve is on the R in 2.2 miles. From Hwy 525 just E of Cultus Bay Rd, turn N onto Surface Rd for 1 mile, then L on Bob Galbreath Rd. Preserve is 0.3 mile on R.*

## ♿ NN. Clinton Beach Park, Clinton (Site 54)

This is the first site in Washington to use full-access beach mats to help people get onto and over sand and as close to water as the tides allow. These mats work for all assistive devices, including canes, walkers, wheelchairs, motorized scooters, and wagons. The Port of South Whidbey and Island Beach Access (**islandbeachaccess.org**) changed or added many amenities in addition to the mats. (Port of South Whidbey)

*Follow directions to Site 54, pg. 97.*

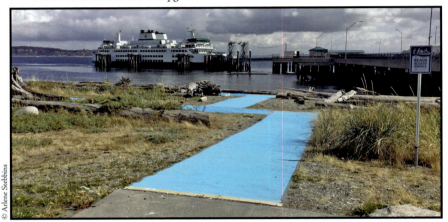

*Clinton Beach Park with ADA mats*

## OO. The Whidbey Institute, Clinton

The public is welcome on the trails of this privately-owned, 106-acre forest and meadow called the Chinook lands, a reserve that protects the headwaters of the Maxwelton Creek watershed. Explore 4½ miles of hilly trails through healthy, mature forest. Open from dawn to dusk, 365 days a year but no bicycles, horses, dogs or other pets are allowed. (The Whidbey Institute)

*6449 Old Pietila Rd. From Hwy 525 at Ken's Korner, turn S onto Cultus Bay Rd. In 0.7 mile turn R on Campbell Rd. In 0.4 mile turn L on Old Pietila Rd at the sign for Whidbey Institute and Chinook Lands. There is parking to the right of the entrance, and two more parking lots 0.4 mile down Old Pietila Road.*

## PP. Hammons Family Farm Preserve, Clinton

Offering an easy walk and panoramic views of Cultus Bay, this 9-acre preserve includes a grassy path over meadows, a stream, and an old orchard. (Whidbey Camano Land Trust)

*7713 Possession Rd. From Hwy 525 at Ken's Korner, go S on Cultus Bay Rd for 4.7 miles. Continue straight onto Possession Rd with parking 300 ft on L.*

## QQ. Possession Point State Park (Site 56)

Steps on the upland side of the parking area lead to a steep trail that ends

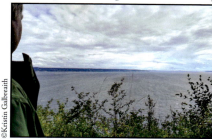

©Kristin Galbreath

*Possession Point State Park view*

nearly a mile later at a 350-foot overlook of Puget Sound. The main trail from the parking lot leads down to the beach. From here, walk south along the beach to see some of Puget Sound's most spectacular bluffs, displaying multiple layers of geologic history. (WA State Parks)

*Follow directions to Site 56, pgs. 99-100.*

## RR. Possession Beach Waterfront Park (Site 57)

The Dorothy Cleveland Trail offers a 1½ mile round trip walk from shore to an elevation of 390 feet. The paved and gravel paths in the park reveal multiple beach and wetland habitats. (Port of South Whidbey)

*Follow directions to Site 57, pg. 101.*

### ♿ RR2. Possession Beach Waterfront Park accessible trail

A firm gravel trail leads to picnic tables near the beach with views over Saratoga Passage and the Mukilteo-Clinton ferry route. Seabirds and the occasional whale can be seen. The habitat includes wild roses, beach wildflowers, marsh plants, and seaside grasses. A wooden bridge crosses the marsh to another trail for closer viewing of the still-water ecology. A slight lip to the bridge may be difficult for wheelchair access.

Trail access is from a parking spot by an "unloading" sign or from handicapped parking nearby. A picnic table and grill are here. The bathroom is designated ADA, but the walkway slope from the handicapped-designated area may be too steep for some in wheelchairs.

*Once in the park, stay to R toward the boat ramp. The handicapped parking is immediately to the left at the beginning of the flat area. The 10-minute unloading spot is a short distance farther toward the beach.*

# TABLE OF SHORELINE ACCESSES

*Section colors correspond with Chapter 3 divisions.*

■ *North Whidbey*   ■ *Central Whidbey*   ■ *South Whidbey*

■ *Camano Island*

● Amenity or activity available.

▲ Barrier-free access to one or more features. May not meet ADA Guidelines.

**Parking:** 1, 2, etc. = Number of spaces. A = Multiple lots. B = No on-site parking, but nearby public parking.

**Accessible amenities:** Triangle = reasonably barrier-free.

**Amenities:** Restroom (flush), pit/portable toilet, potable water, picnic shelters, picnic tables, barbecue grill/fire pit, and playground. (Restrooms may be closed at night, seasonally, for maintenance, or for a variety of reasons.)

**Dock/pier:** Boat dock and/or fishing pier. Some docks removed seasonally.

**Moorage:** Boat moorage. Limitations may apply.

**Boat ramp:** Tides may limit. Some boat-trailer parking.

**Hand-carry boat:** Suitable to hand-carry kayaks, canoes, etc.

**Beach walking:** Connects with 600 feet or more of public tideland.

**Swimming:** Considered good for swimming.

**Fishing:** Shore casting, WDFW permit and seasons apply.

**Bird watching:** More information pages 137-142. See page 155.

**Trails:** Upland trails. Descriptions and ADA accessibility in Chapter 6.

**Parking vista:** View from parking area.

**WWT camp:** Washington Water Trails campsite for those arriving by water in a non-motorized boat.

**Ownership:** CP=Town of Coupeville; DOD = US Department of Defense; EL = Washington State Parks, National Park Service, The Nature Conservancy, and a Sherman-Bishop Farms easement; IC=Island County; LY = City of Langley; OH = City of Oak Harbor; PC = Port of Coupeville; PSW = Port of South Whidbey; PSW/IC = Port of South Whidbey & Island County; SP = Washington State Parks; SWSD = South Whidbey School District; WDFW = Washington Department of Fish & Wildlife (Vehicle Use Permit required).

**Length of public beach:** Estimated length of public tideland reachable from the access before encountering private tideland. None = no tideland. Researched using county property records and descriptions, but we can't guarantee its accuracy.

| Site # | Site Name | Parking | Accessible amenities | Restroom (flush) | Pit/portable toilet | Drinking water | Picnic tables | Picnic shelters | Barbecue/fire pit | Playground | Dock/pier | Moorage | Boat ramp | Hand-carry boat | Beach walking | Swimming | Fishing | Bird watching | Trails | Parking vista | WWT camp | Ownership | Length of public beach |
|---|---|---|---|---|---|---|---|---|---|---|---|---|---|---|---|---|---|---|---|---|---|---|---|
| 1 | Deception Pass State Park | A | ▲ | ▲ | ● | ▲ | ▲ | ▲ | ▲ | ● | ● | ● | | ● | ● | ● | | ● | ▲ | ● | | SP | 14 miles |
| 2 | Cornet Bay County Dock | 10 | | | ● | | | | | | ● | ● | | ● | | | | ● | | ● | | IC | 50 ft. |
| 3 | Cornet Bay Boat Launch | 110 | ▲ | ▲ | | ▲ | ▲ | | ▲ | | ▲ | ● | | ● | ● | | | ● | ▲ | ● | | SP | 2.3 miles |
| 4 | Hoypus Point | 110,6 | | | | | | | | | | | | | | | | ● | ▲ | ● | | SP | 2.3 miles |
| 5 | Ala Spit County Park | 10-15 | | | ● | | | | | | | | | | ● | | | ● | | ● | | IC | 1,187 ft. |
| 6 | Moran Beach | 10-15 | | | ● | | | | | | | | | | ● | | | ● | | ● | ● | IC | 100 ft. |
| 7 | Dugualla Bay Preserve | 8+ | | | | | | | | | | | | | | | | ● | ● | | | WCLT | 1.5 miles |
| 8 | Dugualla State Park | 10 | | | | | | | | | | | | | ● | | | ● | ● | | | SP | 1.3 miles |
| 9 | Borgman Road End | 5 | | | | | | | | | | | | | | | | ● | | ● | | IC | 40 ft. |
| 10 | Mariner's Cove Boat Ramp | 8 | | | | | | | | | | | | ● | | | | ● | | ● | | IC | 245 ft. |
| 11 | Oak Harbor City Marina | 50+ | ▲ | ▲ | ● | ▲ | ▲ | ● | ▲ | ● | ▲ | ● | | ● | ● | | ● | ● | ▲ | ● | | OH | 0.5 mile |
| 12 | Pioneer Way East | B | | | | | | | | | | | | | | | ● | ● | ▲ | ● | | OH | 644 ft. |
| 13 | Flintstone Park | 13+ | ▲ | ▲ | | ▲ | ▲ | ● | | | ● | | | | | | ● | ● | ▲ | ● | | OH | 415 ft. |
| 14 | Windjammer Park | A | ▲ | ▲ | | ▲ | ▲ | ● | ▲ | ▲ | | | | | ● | ● | | ● | ▲ | ● | | OH | 2,100 ft. |
| 15 | Rocky Point (US Navy, restricted) | 20+ | ▲ | | | | | | | ● | | | | | ● | | | ● | | ● | | DOD | 0.5 mile |
| 16 | Joseph Whidbey State Park | 25+ | | | ▲ | ● | ▲ | ● | ● | | | | | | ● | | | ● | ● | ● | | SP | 0.6 mile |
| 17 | West Beach Vista | 10 | | | | | | | | | | | | | ● | | | ● | ● | ● | | IC | 1.8 miles |
| 18 | Hastie Lake County Park | 10 | | | | | | | | | | | | | ● | | | ● | | ● | | IC | 2.4 miles |
| 19 | Monroe Landing | 16 | | | ● | | | | | | | | ● | ● | ● | | | ● | | ● | | IC | 0.5 mile |
| 20 | Libbey Beach Park | 10 | | | ● | | | | ● | | | | ● | ● | ● | | | ● | | ● | | IC | 13 miles |
| 21 | Fort Ebey State Park | A | ▲ | ▲ | | | ▲ | ● | ● | | | | | ● | ● | | ● | ● | ▲ | ● | ● | SP | 13 miles |
| 22 | Grasser's Lagoon | 10-15 | ▲ | | ● | ▲ | ▲ | | ▲ | | | | | ● | ● | | ● | ● | | ● | | WDFW | 0.5 mile |

| Site # | Site Name | Parking | Accessible amenities | Restroom (flush) | Pit/portable toilet | Drinking water | Picnic tables | Picnic shelters | Barbecue/fire pit | Playground | Dock/pier | Moorage | Boat ramp | Hand-carry boat | Beach walking | Swimming | Fishing | Bird watching | Trails | Parking vista | WWT camp | Ownership | Length of public beach |
|---|---|---|---|---|---|---|---|---|---|---|---|---|---|---|---|---|---|---|---|---|---|---|---|
| 23 | Mueller Park | 6-8 | | | | | | | | | | | | ● | ● | | | ● | | ● | | WDFW | 0.9 mile |
| 24 | Coupeville Town Park | 16 | ▲ | ▲ | | | ● | ● | ● | ● | | | | | ● | | | | | | | CP | 0.5 mile |
| 25 | Coupeville Wharf & Beach | B | ▲ | ▲ | | ▲ | ▲ | | | | ▲ | | | | ● | | | ● | | | | PC | 0.5 mile |
| 26 | Captain Coupe Park | 10-12 | ▲ | ▲ | | ● | ▲ | | ▲ | | ● | | | | ● | | | ● | | ● | | CP | 1.6 miles |
| 27 | Long Point | 8-10 | ▲ | | | | | | | | | | | | | ● | | | | ● | | IC | 2.5 miles |
| 28 | Ebey's Landing | 10+ | ▲ | ▲ | ▲ | | ● | | | | | | | | ● | | ● | ● | ▲ | ● | | EL | 7.5 miles |
| 29 | Fort Casey State Park | A | ▲ | ▲ | ▲ | | ▲ | | ● | | | ● | ● | | ● | | ● | ● | | ● | | SP | 2.1 miles |
| 30 | Keystone Jetty | 50+ | | | | ● | ● | | | | | | ● | ● | ● | | ● | ● | | ● | | SP | 500 ft. |
| 31 | Keystone Spit | 50+ | | | | | | | | | | | | ● | ● | | ● | ● | ● | ● | | SP | 1.5 miles |
| 32 | Driftwood Beach Park | 20 | | | ● | | | | | | | | | ● | ● | | | ● | | ● | | IC | 1.5 miles |
| 33 | Ledgewood Beach Access | 5-6 | | | | | | | | | | | | ● | ● | | | ● | | ● | | IC | 2.5 miles |
| 34 | Hidden Beach | 12-14 | | | | | | | | | | | | ● | ● | | | ● | | ● | | IC | 730 ft. |
| 35 | Wonn Rd | 0 | | | | | | | | | | | | ● | | | ● | ● | | | | IC | 25 ft. |
| 36A | Lagoon Point North | 8-10 | | | ● | | | | | | | | | ● | | | ● | ● | | ● | | IC | 397 ft. |
| 36B | Lagoon Point South | 2-3 | | | | | | | | | | | | ● | | | ● | | | | | IC | 30 ft. |
| 37 | South Whidbey State Park | 50 | ▲ | ▲ | ▲ | ▲ | ▲ | ● | ▲ | | | | ● | ● | ● | | ● | ● | ▲ | | | SP | 600 ft. |
| 38 | Bush Point Boat Launch | 12 | ▲ | ▲ | ▲ | ● | ● | | | | ● | | | ● | ● | | | | | | | PSW | 5.7 miles |
| 39 | Bush Point-Sandpiper Rd | 2-4 | | | | | | | | | | | | ● | | | | | | | | IC | 45 ft. |
| 40 | Mutiny Bay Vista | 7 | | | | | | | | | | | | | | | | ● | | | | IC | 295 ft. |
| 41 | Freeland Park | 30+ | ▲ | ▲ | ● | ▲ | ● | ▲ | ▲ | ▲ | ● | ● | | ● | ● | ● | | ● | | ● | | PSW/IC | 0.4 mile |
| 42 | Robinson Park/Mutiny Bay | 30+ | ▲ | | ● | | | | | | | | | ● | ● | | | ● | | ● | | PSW/IC | 360 ft. |
| 43 | Mutiny Bay Shores/Limpet Ln. | 1-2 | | | | ● | | | | | | | | ● | ● | | ● | ● | | | | IC | 950 ft. |
| 44 | Double Bluff Beach | 24 | ▲ | | ▲ | | ● | | | | | | | ● | ● | ● | ● | ● | | ● | | IC | 2 miles |

| Site # | Site Name | Parking | Accessible amenities | Restroom (flush) | Pit/portable toilet | Drinking water | Picnic tables | Picnic shelters | Barbecue/fire pit | Playground | Dock/pier | Moorage | Boat ramp | Hand-carry boat | Beach walking | Swimming | Fishing | Bird watching | Trails | Parking vista | WWT camp | Ownership | Length of public beach |
|---|---|---|---|---|---|---|---|---|---|---|---|---|---|---|---|---|---|---|---|---|---|---|---|
| 45 | Deer Lagoon | 8-10 | | | | | | | | | | | | ● | | | | ● | ● | | | IC | None |
| 46 | Sunlight Beach Accesses | 8-9 | | | | | | | | | | | | ● | | | | ● | | | | IC | 0.3 mile |
| 47 | Lone Lake County Park | 27 | ▲ | | ● | | | | | | | | ● | ● | ● | | ● | ● | | | | WDFW | None |
| 48 | Goss Lake County Park | 8 | | | ● | | | | | | | | ● | ● | | | ● | ● | | | | WDFW | None |
| 49 | Langley Seawall Park | B | | | | | ● | | | | | | | | ● | | ● | ● | | | | LY | 1,000 ft. |
| 50 | South Whidbey Harbor | 10 | ▲ | ▲ | | ▲ | ▲ | | | | ▲ | ● | ● | ● | | ● | ● | ● | | ● | | PSW | 200 ft. |
| 51 | Maxwelton Nature Preserve | 7 | | | ● | | | | | | | | | | | ● | ● | ● | ▲ | | | SWSD | None |
| 52 | Dave Mackie Pk./Maxwelton Bch. | 66 | ▲ | ▲ | ● | ▲ | ▲ | | ▲ | | | | | | | ● | ● | ● | | ● | | PSW/IC | 420 ft. |
| 53 | Deer Lake Park | 6 | ▲ | ▲ | | ▲ | ▲ | ▲ | ▲ | ▲ | | | | ● | | | ● | ● | | | | WDFW | None |
| 54 | Clinton Beach and Pier | 8 | ▲ | ▲ | | ▲ | ● | | ▲ | | ▲ | ● | | | | ● | ● | ● | | | | PSW | 179 ft. |
| 55 | Glendale Beach Preserve | 11 | ▲ | | ● | | ▲ | | | | | | | ● | | | ● | ● | | | | WCLT | 420 ft. |
| 56 | Possession Point State Park | 10 | | | | | | | | | | | ● | | ● | | ● | ● | ● | ● | ● | SP | 0.9 mile |
| 57 | Possession Beach Park | 30+ | ▲ | ▲ | ● | ▲ | ▲ | | ▲ | | ● | | ● | ● | ● | | ● | ● | ▲ | ● | | PSW | 677 ft. |
| 58 | English Boom Preserve | 14 | ▲ | | | | | ▲ | | | | | | ● | | | | ● | ▲ | ● | | IC | 300 ft. |
| 59 | Utsalady Beach | 10 | | | ● | | ● | | | | | | | ● | | | | ● | | | | IC | 380 ft. |
| 60 | Utsalady Vista Park | 4 | | | | | ● | | ● | | | | | ● | | | | | | ● | | IC | None |
| 61 | Maple Grove Park | 18 | | | ● | ● | ● | | | | | | ● | ● | | | | | | | | IC | 250 ft. |
| 62 | Livingston Bay | 10-15 | | | | | | | | | | | | | | | | ● | | | | IC | 90 ft. |
| 63 | Iverson Spit Preserve | 10+ | | | ● | | ● | | | | | | | | ● | | ● | ● | ● | ● | | IC | 0.5 mile |
| 64 | Cavalero Park | 15-20 | | | ● | | ● | | | | | | | | | ● | | ● | | | | IC | 250 ft. |
| 65 | Cama Beach State Park | A | ▲ | ▲ | | ▲ | ▲ | | | | | | ● | ● | ● | ● | ● | ● | ● | ● | ● | SP | 1.1 miles |
| 66 | Camano Island State Park | A | ▲ | ▲ | | ▲ | ▲ | ▲ | ▲ | | | | | ● | ● | ● | ● | ● | ● | | | SP | 1.2 miles |
| 67 | Tillicum Beach | 4 | | | | | ● | | | | | | | ● | ● | ● | ● | ● | | | | IC | 80 ft. |
| 68 | Barnum Point County Park | 19+ | | | ● | | | | | | | | | | ● | ● | ● | ● | | | | IC | 1 mile |

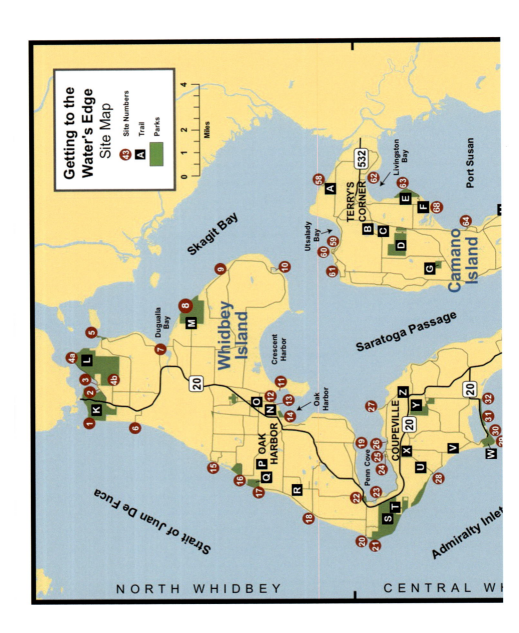

Getting to the
Water's Edge
Site Map

43 Site Numbers
A Trail
Parks

0 1 2 4
Miles

Skagit Bay

Utsalady Bay

532

Livingston Bay

Port Susan

TERRY'S CORNER

58 A
62
63
E
F
68
59
60
61
B
C
D
G
64

Camano Island

9
10
8 M

Duqualla Bay

Whidbey Island

Crescent Harbor

Saratoga Passage

5
7
4a L
4b
3
2
K
1
6

20
11
12
13
O
N
14
Oak Harbor

27

COUPEVILLE
Z
Y
20
32
31
30
29

15
16
17
Q P OAK HARBOR
R
19
25 26
24 23
22
Penn Cove
X
U
V
28
W

18
S T
20
21

Strait of Juan De Fuca

Admiralty Inlet

NORTH WHIDBEY          CENTRAL WH

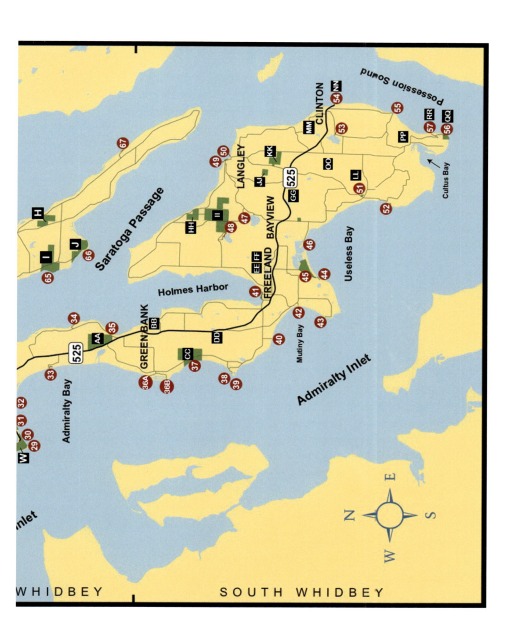

# INDEX

## SPONSORS AND PARTNERS
## Thank you to all our generous Sponsors and Partners whose financial support funded the printing of this book!

### Member Supporters ($100-)

Anonymous (Three)
Jeanne Amundsen and Kurt Herzog
Joani Boose
Cheryl and Bill Bradkin
David and Linda Brubaker
Jack and Peg Burchard
Scott and Marietta Cole

Margaret Marshall
Vanessa Meriwether Irvine
Sarah Schmidt and Bill Rick
Wendy and Mark Visconty
Tom and Sharon Vos
John Welsch and Ellen Molbak Welsch

### Member Sponsors ($250+)

**The Whidbey Sound Water Stewards class of 2019** extends heartfelt gratitude to Nancy Neudecker, Lee Badovinus, Mary Ann Imkamp, and Scott Cole for their inspiring facilitation of the life-changing programs presented in SWS training. Their dedication, professionalism, and passion continues by empowering each of us with the knowledge, skills, and opportunities to make positive contributions toward the betterment of the planet.

**Anonymous:** In memory of Connie Clark, Beach Watcher (class of 2007) and Sound Water Steward extraordinaire.

**Anonymous:** I journeyed to Whidbey and found home. The wonderful people of Sound Water Stewards have welcomed me home and now *Getting to the Water's Edge* is showing me how to explore my home. Thank you Sound Water Stewards.

**Lee Badovinus:** "Our task must be to free ourselves… by widening our circle of compassion to embrace all living creatures and the whole of nature and its beauty." -- Albert Einstein

**PB invites you to:** Go to the beach! Explore, enjoy and cherish.

**Dave Davis and Barbara Hardman:** Driving the length of Whidbey Island are amazing bucolic vistas, but one is only teased with glimpses of its miles of prime shoreline. In this book, Sound Water Stewards guide us to those places where we can discover the Island edge and its treasures trove that await us.

**Kristin and Scott Galbreaith:** Honoring Helen Johnson Collins and Natalie Tengwald Galbreaith for their love of nature, education, and the Pacific Northwest.

**Bonnie Gretz:** Thank you to Sound Water Stewards of Island County for putting this wonderful community resource together, an all-volunteer effort! When I first moved to Whidbey Island in 2011, the edition then available was very helpful to me as I learned about my new home. Sound Water Stewards of Island County is one of the best assets of Whidbey and Camano Islands!

**Libby Hayward:** SWS Class of 2004, Whidbey Audubon Society, Windermere Real Estate. As a real estate broker, I enjoy giving clients *Getting to the Water's Edge* as a closing gift and welcome the new and expanded version. Thanks to all who contributed to this remarkable field guide for all who love, appreciate and respect our phenomenal beaches! 360-678-6677, libby@whidbey.com

**Jill Hein:** This book is a wonderful resource for recreationists and fishermen – and a GREAT asset for land based whale watchers – we all want to see our iconic whales whenever possible. orcanetwork.org

**Donald and Joyce Leak** became Beach Watchers in 2002 after moving to Camano in 1998. They learned lots about Island County and met new friends. Donald served as chair of the Beach Watchers Board of Directors. He also served on the committee that helped Beach Watchers evolve to Sound Water Stewards.

Trent Lowe

Andrea Malott

**Jeanie and Paul Ben McElwain:** To all our world's volunteers who stand by our waters—one foot in grief and the other in celebration—and ask "What can I do now?" Who step into the answer and carry on. To love our earth and seas so deeply in these times is an act of Courage. Thank you.

Nancy Neudecker

Charles Seablom

Kestutis & Birute Tautvydas

## Community Sponsors ($250)

**Boatyard Inn** invites you to enjoy waterfront lodging and the sea a few feet from your private deck. Wake to spectacular views of Saratoga Passage and the Cascades. Take advantage of direct access to Langley's picturesque marina, whale watching and kayaking. Walk to Langley by the Sea with restaurants, galleries, shops, and much more. Find us at boatyardinn.com.

**Cairn Financial,** located in Langley would like to extend our heartfelt thanks to the SWS volunteers for all they do.

**Donna King, Cama Beach Café & Catering,** camabeachcafe.com. Located in the Great Hall overlooking Puget Sound in Cama Beach State Park, 1880 SW Camano Dr, Camano Island, WA 98282. Open 8-2 Daily in summer; in the off-season from 8-2 Fridays-Sundays. Donna King's delicious creations feature healthy fresh food. Named one of the top ten brunch restaurants by Best of Washington.

**Camano Island Chamber of Commerce** promotes economic vitality, partnering with businesses and the community to grow our unique island culture. The Camano Island Chamber of Commerce is the pulse of our community. By working together and embracing innovative ways to expand people's ideas, we will secure our future and build a better community for generations to live, work, and enjoy.

**Friends of Camano Island Parks** is a non-profit 501(c)(3) all-volunteer Camano Island organization. Our mission is to preserve, protect, acquire, and provide stewardship for the public properties on Camano Island. We maintain trails and infrastructure at 14 public properties covering 1600 acres with over 20 miles of trails. Our 30 active volunteers provide thousands of hours of labor each year.

**Dan Gulden, Broker,** John L Scott Whidbey Island South, 216 First Street, Langley, WA 98260, 206-854-3150, DanG@johnlscott.com. "The sea, once it casts its spell, holds one in its net of wonder forever." – Jacques Yves Cousteau

**Island Beach Access** is a charitable organization whose mission is to identify, enhance, and preserve beach access on Whidbey Island for current and future generations while respecting both public and private interests. We welcome your questions, concerns, and support! Please support us with donations to Whidbey Island Land and Shore Trust, our 501(c)(3) non-profit parent.

**Orca Network's Langley Whale Center** celebrates and shares the lives of gray whales, orcas, and other marine mammals of the Salish Sea. Wander through the world of whales at 105 Anthes Ave. in Langley to learn from exhibits, our interactive Ocean Listening booth, and marine mammal specimens collected and prepared by our Central Puget Sound Stranding Network. Free Admission.

**Orca Network** is a non-profit organization dedicated to raising awareness of the whales of the Pacific Northwest and the importance of providing them healthy and safe habitats. Orca Network finds ways for people to work together to protect the rich, beautiful, diverse habitats and inhabitants of the Salish Sea. Orca Network–Connecting whales and people in the Pacific Northwest.

**Camano Center's 2nd Chance Thrift Shop**, through the sale of gently used donations of household items, provides financial support for the programs and services the Camano Center provides to our seniors and community. In addition, we give our donors a great way to help reduce their impact on the landfill and our customers a greener shopping experience. camanocenter.org or 2ndchancethriftshop.org.

**The Rotary Club of Stanwood/Camano Island**, through fellowship, diversity, discovery, and partnership is dedicated to engaging the community while having fun and making a positive impact on the lives of those we serve, both locally and globally.

**Whidbey Camano Land Trust** permanently preserves, restores, and cares for our naturally beautiful islands to keep them the way you love. Natural areas. Local family farms. Wildlife habitat. Scenic vistas. Clean water and air. And, trails and beach access connecting people to nature. As a nonprofit, we're supported by private donations. Visit us at wclt.org.

**Whidbey Watershed Stewards** is a non-profit organization. We proactively and holistically foster environmental responsibility through education, research, and restoration. We offer inspirational educational experiences at the Maxwelton Outdoor Classroom for K-5 students, field courses for 6-8 students. As educators we engage the community with public presentations, habitat surveys, restoration work parties, and more. Facilitating educational experiences, we foster environmental stewardship.

### *Partner Sponsors ($500)*

**A.S.E.&T. Landsurveying:** Thank you to the volunteers.

**Cama Beach Foundation** is a nonprofit organization that operates with an all-volunteer staff. Our goal is to support Camano Island State Park and Cama Beach Historical State Park by offering visitors educational and interpretive programs that enhance their visits. Cama Beach Foundation operations are funded by generous donations and by proceeds from sales at the historic Cama Beach Store.

**Inn at Langley, Matt Costello**, Hotel General Manager and Chef.

**Candace Jordan, Realtor,** 206-391-0189, cjordan@whidbey.com, CandaceJordanTeam. com. Whether you are buying, selling or dreaming, I'm committed to helping you realize your real estate goals on Whidbey Island. I trust you'll find me knowledgeable, enthusiastic, professional and a good listener! Let's meet at the water's edge!

**Dana MacInnis, Realtor,** John L Scott Whidbey Island South. 360-914-0685 danam@ johnlscott.com. Compassionate service with a backbone of integrity. I consider myself a steward of people and place, bringing a unique combination of deep listening and fierce advocacy to my clients. "Tell me, what it is that you plan to do with your one wild and precious life?" – Mary Oliver

**Lisa Rogers, Broker,** 216 First St, Langley WA 98260, 360-929-5968, lisa@whidbeyisland.com, http://lisa@whidbey-island.com, lisar.johnlscott.com. "We are tied to the ocean. And when we go back to the sea, whether it is to sail or to watch – we are going back from whence we came." – John F. Kennedy

**Karen White, Realtor,** 216 First St, Langley, 360-544-2380; karenwhite@johnlscott. com, karenwhite.johnlscott.com. "I've learned that people will forget what you said, people will forget what you did, but people will never forget how you made them feel." – Maya Angelou. I look forward to making your Whidbey Island real estate experience one you will remember and feel good about for years to come.